# Phlebotomy
# Handbook

# Phlebotomy Handbook

**Diana Garza, M.S, M.T.(ASCP), C.L.S.(NCA)**
Senior Education Coordinator and Instructor
Program in Medical Technology
School of Allied Health Sciences
University of Texas Health Science Center
Texas Medical Center
Houston, Texas

**Kathleen Becan-McBride, Ed.D., M.T.(ASCP), C.L.S.(NCA)**
Program Director and Associate Professor
Program in Medical Technology
School of Allied Health Sciences
Associate Professor–Department of Pathology and Laboratory Medicine, Medical School
Associate Professor–Graduate School of Biomedical Sciences
University of Texas Health Science Center
Texas Medical Center
Houston, Texas

**APPLETON-CENTURY-CROFTS/Norwalk, Connecticut**

0-8385-7843-8

85 86 87 88 / 10 9 8 7 6 5 4 3 2

Prentice-Hall International, Inc., London
Prentice-Hall of Australia, Pty. Ltd., Sydney
Prentice-Hall Canada, Inc.
Prentice-Hall of India Private Limited, New Delhi
Prentice-Hall of Japan, Inc., Tokyo
Prentice-Hall of Southeast Asia (Pte.) Ltd., Singapore
Whitehall Books Ltd., Wellington, New Zealand
Editora Prentice-Hall do Brasil Ltda., Rio de Janeiro

**Library of Congress Cataloging in Publication Data**
Garza, Diana.
  Phlebotomy handbook.
  Includes index.
  1. Bloodletting—Handbooks, manuals, etc. I. Becan-
McBride, Kathleen, 1949-    . II Title. [DNLM:
1. Bloodletting—Handbooks.   WB 39 P573]
RM 182.G37   1984      616.07'561      84-3101
ISBN 0-8385-7843-8

Design: Jean M. Sabato

PRINTED IN THE UNITED STATES OF AMERICA

*To my husband Peter McLaughlin and my parents*
*for their affection and constant support.*

D.G.


*To my husband Mark, sons Patrick and Jonathan,*
*parents, and parents-in-law*
*for their support and devotion.*

K. B.-McB.

# Contributors

**Pamela B. Bollinger, B.S., M.T.(ASCP)**
Chief Technologist, Hematology, Department of Laboratory Medicine, University of Texas System Cancer Center, M. D. Anderson Hospital and Tumor Institute, Houston, Texas

**Carrie D. Brailas, B.S., M.T.(ASCP)**
Assistant Chief Technologist, Hematology, Department of Laboratory Medicine, University of Texas System Cancer Center, M. D. Anderson Hospital and Tumor Institute, Houston, Texas

**Amelia T. Carr, B.S., M.T.(ASCP), C.L.S.(NCA)**
Phlebotomy Instructor/Coordinator, School of Allied Health Sciences, University of Texas Health Science Center, Houston, Texas

**Karen Hlavaty, M.T.(ASCP), C.L.S.(NCA)**
Assistant Supervisor–Hematology, Department of Pathology and Laboratory Medicine, Hermann Hospital, Houston, Texas

**Annot F. Littlepage, Ed.D., M.T.(ASCP), C.L.S.(NCA)**
Assistant Professor, Program in Medical Technology; Associate Director of the Clinical Laboratories for Educational Services, University of Texas Medical Branch, Galveston, Texas

**Doris L. Ross, Ph.D., M.T.(ASCP), C.L.S.(NCA)**
Associate Dean and Professor, School of Allied Health Sciences; Professor, Department of Pathology and Laboratory Medicine, Medical School; Professor, Graduate School Biomedical Sciences, University of Texas Health Science Center, Houston, Texas

# Contents

# Preface

The aim of this book is to provide practical instruction and advice to the beginning as well as the more experienced person performing specimen collection. Because of the expansion of diagnostic technology in the field of clinical laboratory medicine, the volume of laboratory procedures has increased greatly. As a result, the proper collection of patient specimens has become vitally important. Specimen collection requires knowledge of equipment and proper techniques as well as quality assurance procedures, interpersonal skills, professional liability and health-care institutional safety requirements. All of these essential topics are covered in this handbook.

This book developed from our perception that students beginning to collect specimens and persons already advanced in performing and managing specimen collection needed practical information. Thus, we offer recommendations for improving laboratory testing and reporting, and ultimately, for providing superior patient care.

We are indebted to many individuals for assistance in preparing this textbook. We would like to express appreciation to Bill Fetter, David Payne, Barbara Nemitz, Debra Hines, Jim Hixon with Becton-Dickinson Vacutainer Systems, Bob McEwen with Ulster Scientific, Inc., Tuyet-Van Phung, Lydia Morris, Inga Danville with the Hermann Hospital Blood Bank, Peggy McCall and Helen Harrell with Hermann Hospital, Ann Cork with M. D. Anderson Hospital, Pam Chamallas from Beckman Instruments, Martin Valaske, and Gordon Briggs, the College of American Pathology, and Coulter Electronics.

Appreciation is due to the University of Texas School of Allied Health Sciences, Hermann Hospital, the University of Texas Cancer Center M. D. Anderson Hospital and Tumor Institute for a supportive atmosphere during the writing of this book.

We are indebted to our families for enduring the many hours spent developing this book.

# CHAPTER 1

# Phlebotomy and the Health-Care Setting

Kathleen Becan-McBride

## INTRODUCTION TO PHLEBOTOMY

The development of new diagnostic techniques, clinical laboratory technology, and automated instruments has greatly increased the volume of laboratory testing. As a result, a member of the clinical laboratory team, the "phlebotomist," has emerged with a greater role in facilitating the specimen collection process. The main function for this vital laboratory member is to obtain patients' blood specimens by venipuncture and microcollection techniques and to facilitate collection and transportation of other clinical laboratory specimens.

In the past, phlebotomists were trained on a one-to-one basis as part of on-the-job training. However, due to the increase in laboratory assays and need for quality assurance in laboratory test results, many colleges, universities, and hospitals have implemented phlebotomy curricula to prepare individuals to assume the responsibilities and tasks of phlebotomists. Consequently, the field of phlebotomy has expanded, and the phlebotomist now is an integral member of the health-care team.

## THE HEALTH-CARE TEAM IN HOSPITALS AND CLINICS

Clinical laboratories are located in various types of settings and institutions. Clinical laboratories with the highest level of technologic and organizational complexity are usually in hospitals; and consequently, that is where many phlebotomists work. Hospitals are classified in different ways. For example, one type of classification referred to as "clinical" is based on the type of patients treated. Clinical hospitals include general types that serve patients with various illnesses and special-care hospitals are those that treat only a few types of illnesses. Included in special-care classification are pediatrics, cancer, maternity, and psychiatric hospitals.

Another type of classification for hospitals pertains to the type of ownership or control (government or nongovernment). Within the governmental classification are federal hospitals such as the Veterans Administration hospitals, military hospitals, and the United States Public Health Service hospitals. Other types of governmental hospitals include state, county, and city facilities. Governmental hospitals have a public tax base for support of health-care facilities.

Nongovernmental hospitals differ in ownership and thus, control. For example, the largest group of nongovernmental hospitals are referred to as community hospitals because they are owned by the community. The governing board has representatives from the community and relates the needs of the community to the hospital. Other types of nongovernmental hospitals include church hospitals and privately-owned hospitals.

Hospital size is commonly designated by the number of inpatients and outpatients seen per day. Another measurement is the number of beds the hospital contains. This bed number may be recorded as adult beds and/or pediatric beds.

Other examples of health-care facilities in which phlebotomists may be employed include Health Maintenance Organizations (HMOs), multiphasic screening centers, neighborhood health centers, and medical group practices. An HMO is a comprehensive group practice center financed by prepayment or regular monthly accounts. Facilities are usually integrated with the hospital, screening center, clinic and physician's offices located in one central area. The multiphasic screening centers have laboratory, radiologic, and electrocardiographic screening examinations for preventive medicine and early detection of disease. The neighborhood health centers offer services to the community and are supported to a great extent by federal money. Most of these centers are located in low income areas and treat and diagnose members of the community on an ambulatory basis. Medical group practices usually consist of physicians, nurses, and other health professionals offering medical care to individuals in need of diagnosis and treatment. The services may be general or specific, depending upon the practice group.

Phlebotomists are employed in all of these health-care institutions. Because each institution has its own philosophy, rules, and regulations, the phlebotomist must become familiar with them in order to perform in the manner expected.

# DEPARTMENTS WITHIN THE HEALTH-CARE SETTING

The rapid scientific advances in diagnostic and treatment instrumentation within health-care settings has led to numerous departments with which the phlebotomist must interact. Within the hospital setting, the phlebotomist should be familiar with radiology, nuclear medicine, radiation therapy, occupational therapy, physical therapy, electrocardiography, encephalography, pharmacy, and of course, the clinical laboratory.

## Radiology

The radiology department uses ionizing radiation for treating disease, fluoroscopic and radiographic x-ray instrumentation for diagnosing, and radioactive isotopes for both diagnosing and treating (Fig. 1-1).

Almost every patient admitted to a hospital (inpatient or outpatient) or to another health-care facility usually becomes a patient in the department of radiology at some time during his or her stay. In radiology, patients and employees must be protected against unnecessary irradiation from radiologic instrumentation. On occasion, the phlebotomist may have to go to the radiology department in order to collect laboratory specimens from the patient. Thus, the phlebotomist should become acquainted with the location and safety requirements of this department.

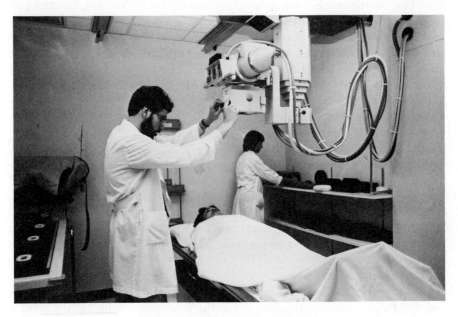

**Figure 1-1.** Photo of x-ray equipment.

Radiology studies sometimes require that the patient be injected with dye. If the phlebotomist finds that the patient has received radiology dyes prior to blood collection, he or she should communicate the patient's name and possible dye interference to the clinical laboratory supervisor in charge of specimen control. The supervisor then can communicate with the laboratory director, clinical pathologist, and attending physician to determine if the dye will interfere in the requested laboratory assays.

## Nuclear Medicine

The nuclear medicine department uses radioactive materials in the diagnosis and treatment of patients and in the study of the disease process. This department is used primarily in diagnosis, and in procedures requiring introduction of a radiotracer into the patient, usually by intravenous injection. The resulting emitted rays are detected by sensitive crystals on the complex instrumentation, which provide sequential imaging and graphic representation of radioactivity. The nuclear medicine procedures differ from radiology predominantly in that the latter use rays transmitted through the patient whereas the former utilize radiation emitted from the patient, resulting in images that provide more anatomic than functional information. As in radiology, the phlebotomist should acquaint him or herself with the location and safety requirements of the nuclear medicine department.

The radioisotopes, which are introduced into a patient for nuclear medicine studies, may interfere in laboratory assays. Thus, the phlebotomist who finds that the patient from whom he or she must collect blood is not in the hospital room but rather in the nuclear medicine department should ask employees in nuclear medicine if the patient has already had a radioisotopic injection. If so, the phlebotomist should report this information to the specimen control supervisor who will then follow-up to determine if the injection will interfere with laboratory assays.

## Radiation Therapy

The department of radiation therapy applies high energy x-rays, cobalt, elution, and other types of radiation in the treatment of disease—especially cancer (Fig. 1-2). The instrumentation used in radiation therapy presents a problem of irradiation greater than that of the radiology department. Thus, safety precautions against unnecessary irradiation are extremely important for patients and employees.

## Occupational Therapy

The department of occupational therapy helps the patient to become as independently active as feasible within the limitations of his or her mental or physical problem. The occupational therapist collaborates with other health professionals (i.e., social workers, nursing staff, attending physician,

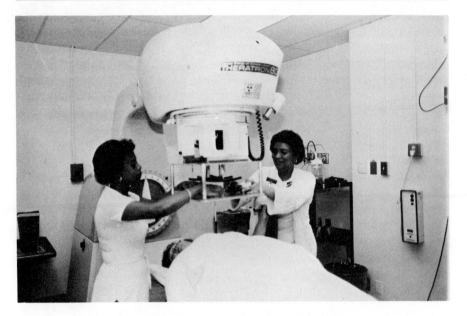

**Figure 1-2.** Photo of radiation therapy equipment.

physical therapist) to plan a therapeutic program of rehabilitating activities for the patient.

Since the patient may spend a considerable amount of time in the occupational therapy department, the phlebotomist should become aware of this department's location if he or she must collect blood from patients who have been taken to this department to undergo therapy.

## Physical Therapy

The role of the physical therapy department is to eliminate the patient's disability or to restore as completely as possible his or her mental or physical abilities that have been impaired by illness or injury (Fig. 1-3). Rehabilitation within this department requires the use of heat, cold, water exercise, ultrasound and/or electricity, and other physical techniques to restore useful activity. Because the rehabilitative service to the patient is usually quite extensive and time consuming, the phlebotomist may, on occasion, need to collect specimens in the physical therapy department.

## Encephalography and Electrocardiography

Another department that the phlebotomist should become aware of is the encephalography department. The electroencephalograph (EEG) is an instrument that records brain waves. It is a sensitive instrument, and therefore the patient must be taken to a special shielded area that is protected against outside electrical or static interference.

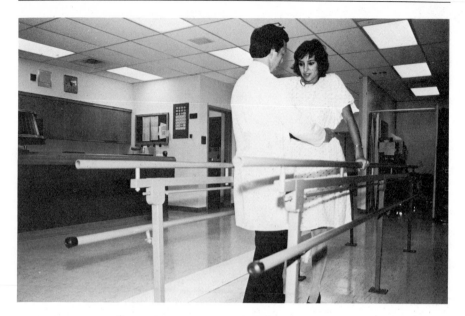

**Figure 1-3.** Photo of physical therapist and patient.

The department of electrocardiography is used as a diagnostic service for the patient. The electrocardiograph (ECG or EKG) records the electric current produced by the contractions of the heart muscle and is used to assist in the diagnosis of heart disease or indicate progress in recovery from heart disease.

### Pharmacy

Almost everyone knows that the pharmacist dispenses medications ordered by a physician. However, in addition, the pharmacist is involved with members of the health-care team as a primary consultant on drug therapy. On many occasions, the pharmacist must communicate with clinical laboratory personnel concerning a patient's blood level of a certain drug when the patient is on drug therapy. In order to monitor therapeutic drug levels, the blood specimens must be drawn at certain time intervals. The phlebotomist may have the responsibility to collect the blood specimens for therapeutic drug monitoring and may need to communicate with the pharmacy department on time intervals of the blood collections.

## DEPARTMENT OF CLINICAL LABORATORY MEDICINE

The rapid advances in clinical laboratory automation and procedures are reflected in the fact that the clinical laboratory has grown faster in past years than has hospital growth in general. Sophisticated technology and automation have provided new dimensions in the diagnosis and treatment of disease.

The clinical laboratory department is composed of two major areas. In the clinical pathology area, blood and other types of body fluids and tissues (such as urine, cerebrospinal fluid (CSF), biopsy specimens and gastric secretions) are analyzed (Fig. 1-4). The area of anatomic pathology is involved in the performance of autopsies, cytology, and surgical pathology procedures. The clinical laboratory is primarily interested in patient services, but is also usually involved in research and development, and teaching in order to assure high quality of laboratory service.

## Clinical Laboratory Personnel

*Laboratory Directors.* The laboratory personnel are frequently directed by a pathologist as shown in the organizational structure of Figure 1-5. The organizational structure of the clinical laboratory is constantly being revised as shown in Figure 1-6 in which the personnel are directed by a complementary relationship between the pathologist and administrative technologist.

The pathologist is a physician who usually has extensive education in pathology (the study and diagnosis of diseases through the utilization of laboratory test results). He or she directs the physician–patient services of the clinical laboratory and has the following responsibilities[1]: assists in the establishment of policies and test protocols; provides consultation services concerning laboratory results to medical–dental staff; teaches continuing

**The Clinical Laboratory as a Subsystem of the Envionment**

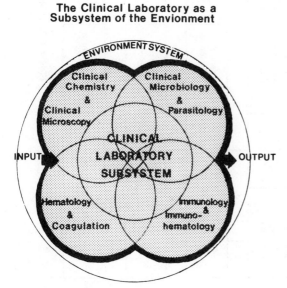

**Figure 1-4.** Clinical laboratory areas.

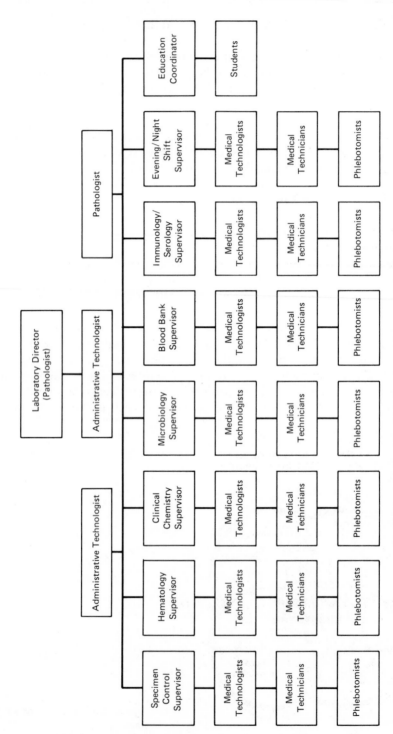

**Figure 1-5.** Organizational structure of a typical clinical laboratory.

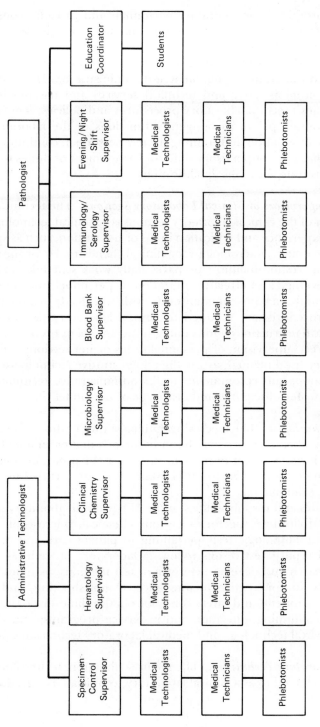

**Figure 1-6.** Organizational structure becoming increasingly common in clinical laboratories.

education programs for laboratory personnel; and provides consultation and interpretation on surgical and autopsy tissues, cytologic specimens and bone marrows.

The administrative technologist is a medical technologist who has had additional education in management and administration. He or she is the director of administrative and technical services and has the following responsibilities[1]: sets up laboratory procedures and policies; employs laboratory personnel; performs budgetary functions of the laboratory; and provides for orientation and training of new personnel, continuing education of technical and supervisory staff, and assignment of duties to personnel commensurate with their qualifications.

***Technical Supervisors of Clinical Laboratory Sections.*** The technical supervisor in each of the clinical laboratory sections is a medical technologist with additional experience and education in his or her section, such as specimen control, hematology, microbiology, or clinical chemistry. He or she assumes the following responsibilities[1]: prepares daily work schedules to provide adequate coverage and effective utilization of personnel; maintains levels of supplies and reagents commensurate with workload; insures that policies and procedures are followed by clinical laboratory personnel; provides technical instructions and training of personnel in his or her section; provides direct supervision of personnel in his or her section; maintains a current procedural manual; assists the administrative technologist in budget preparation; and recommends to the administrative technologist the selection, transfer, discipline, and discharge of personnel.

***Medical Technologist.*** The medical technologist (MT), who is also referred to as clinical laboratory scientist, has a bachelor's degree in a biologic science, which includes a year or more of study in a MT program. Some states have licensing examinations for MTs. Many MTs are certified by national certification examinations.

The duties and responsibilities of the MT (clinical laboratory scientist) include the following[2]: performs various chemical, microscopic, microbiologic, or immunologic tests pertaining to patient care and diagnosis; records and reports test results following laboratory procedures; participates in research and development of new test methods; assumes a major responsibility for preventive maintenance, troubleshooting, and quality control of instruments and safety conditions in the clinical laboratory; participates in continuing education and in-service programs; and assists in teaching medical technology and medical laboratory technician students.

***Medical Laboratory Technician.*** The medical laboratory technician (MLT), who is also referred to as a clinical laboratory technician, is a graduate of a

2-year certificate or associate degree MLT program. Some states require licensing for the MLT and have a licensing examination for this category. Many medical laboratory technicians are certified by MLT or CLT national certification examinations.

Under supervision by a MT or technical supervisor, the MLT performs routine tests and procedures in any assigned laboratory department. He or she records and reports results following laboratory procedures and reports abnormal results to the supervisor. Other duties and responsibilities include: prepares specimens for reference laboratories; prepares reagents as needed; draws blood as required; observes safety procedures and maintains laboratory area and equipment; and participates in continuing education and in-service programs.[2]

***Phlebotomist.*** The phlebotomist is usually required to be a high school graduate or equivalent to enter phlebotomy training. The training varies from one health-care center to another and may take from a few weeks to months, depending on the institution. The phlebotomist may become certified by passing a national certification examination.

Under supervision of the specimen control technical supervisor, the phlebotomist has the following typical duties and responsibilities[3]:

1. collects adequate and correct blood specimens by venipuncture or microtechnique on adults, children, and infants;
2. follows departmental policies to correctly identify the patient before any blood specimen is drawn and to correctly label all specimens drawn;
3. at all times shows concern for and understanding of the patient and promotes the comfort and well-being of the patient as much as possible while performing collecting duties. Patience and persistence are needed when dealing with patients from whom blood specimens are difficult to obtain;
4. starts glucose tolerance procedures and collects remaining specimens at required times. Draws other timed specimens as indicated;
5. picks up and delivers to the laboratory a variety of clinical specimens other than blood;
6. sorts and processes specimens received in central specimen receipt area of department. Maintains orderly and timely flow of specimens to the technical areas;
7. maintains accurate and orderly log records and worksheets where required according to established departmental and hospital protocol;
8. projects an image of professionalism in appearance and conduct at all times.

## Clinical Laboratory Sections

*Clinical Chemistry.* The clinical chemistry section is one of the largest areas in the clinical laboratory. Here, the laboratory procedures that are run (Table 1-1) include the quantitative measurement of serum proteins, blood glucose, serum lipids (triglycerides, cholesterol), serum iron and iron binding levels, serum electrolytes (sodium, potassium, bicarbonate, and chloride), blood gases ($PO_2$, $PCO_2$ pH), serum creatinine, blood urea nitrogen, vitamins (i.e., ascorbic acid, vitamin $B_{12}$, folic acid), enzymes (i.e., lactate dehydrogenase, alanine aminotransferase, creatine phosphate). Also, the clinical chemistry section usually has a toxicology area for drug analysis and an area for the analysis of hormones. Other procedures generally included in clinical chemistry are bilirubin and liver function analysis and cerebrospinal (CSF) and gastric fluid analysis.

The clinical chemistry section has become highly automated, and thus, most of the chemical procedures use less patient's blood for each analysis than in the past. Automation has greatly increased the efficiency and quality assurance within the clinical chemistry section (Fig. 1-7).

*Hematology.* The hematology section is concerned with laboratory assays used to identify diseases of blood-forming tissues. In addition, other processes can be evaluated through changes in the blood. Coagulation, clinical microscopy, and urinalysis are frequently housed in the hematology section. Hematologic results are extremely valuable diagnostic tools and are an integral part of a patient's examination. Most health-care facilities require that the hematologic assay referred to as the complete blood count (CBC) be run on every individual admitted as a patient to the health-care facility. The five components of the CBC are:

1. red blood cell count (RBC);
2. white blood cell count (WBC);
3. hemoglobin (Hgb or Hb);
4. hematocrit (Hct or Crit); and
5. differential white count (Diff).

Other assays evaluated in the hematology section include: reticulocyte count, erythrocyte sedimentation rate (ESR), erythrocyte indices (MCV, MCH, and MCHC). Many of these assays are automated and can simultaneously test a blood specimen for various hematologic parameters (Fig. 1-8). Also, these hematologic instruments can electronically compute results for these assays.

Coagulation tests, usually performed in the hematology section, are run to determine the clotting ability of the blood. The two most common coagulation assays are prothrombin time (PT) and partial thromboplastin time (PTT). Screening tests and confirmatory assays for classical hemo-

**TABLE 1-1. A SUMMARY OF MAJOR TESTS PERFORMED IN THE CLINICAL LABORATORY SECTIONS**

**Clinical Chemistry Procedures:**
  Total proteins
  Serum protein electrophoresis
  Glucose and glucose tolerance
  Triglycerides
  Cholesterol
  Iron
  Total iron binding capacity (IBC) or (TIBC)
  Electrolytes [sodium ($Na^+$), potassium ($K^+$), chloride ($Cl^-$), bicarbonate ($HCO^-_3$)]
  Magnesium
  Blood gases (pH, $Pco_2$, $Po_2$)
  Creatinine
  Blood urea nitrogen (BUN)
  Uric acid
  Enzymes [e.g., lactate dehydrogenase (LH), alanine aminotransferase (ALT), creatine phosphate (CK)]
  Drug analysis (e.g., gentamicin, tobramycin, primidone, phenytoin, digoxin, quinidine, salicylates, blood alcohol, barbiturate)
  Bilirubin
  Hormones [e.g., thyroxine ($T_4$), insulin, testosterone, renin activity, luteinizing hormone, parathyroid hormone, prolactin, cortisol]

**Clinical Microbiology Procedures:**

| | | |
|---|---|---|
| Acid-fast bacilli (AFB) smear | Fungus direct smear | Ova and parasites |
| Anaerobic culture | GC culture | Pinworm preparation |
| Culture and sensitivity | Gram stain | Stool culture |
| AFB culture | Occult blood | Strep screen |
| Fungus culture | Nose/throat culture | Urine culture |
| Blood culture | | |

**Hematology and Coagulation Procedures:**

| | | |
|---|---|---|
| CSF cell count | Hemoglobin | RBC |
| Differential | Hemoprofile | Reticulocyte count |
| Eosinophil count | LE cell preparation | Sedimentation rate |
| Fecal leukocyte | Nasal eosinophil | Sickle cell preparation |
| Hematocrit | Platelet count | WBC |
| CBC | Partial thromboplastin time | Thrombin time |
| Fibrin split product | Prothrombin time | |
| Fibrinogen | | |

**Clinical Microscopy and Urinalysis Procedures:**

| | Routine UA | | |
|---|---|---|---|
| Hemosiderin | | | Synovial fluid analysis |
| Pregnancy test | pH | Bilirubin | Seminal fluid analysis |
| | Specific gravity | Nitrates | |
| | Protein | Urobilinogen | |
| | Sugar | Ascorbic acid | |
| | Ketones | Occult blood | |

**Immunohematology procedures:**

| | | |
|---|---|---|
| ABO and Rho (D) Type | Antibody SCR indirect | Rh phenotype and genotype |
| ABO Group | Coombs | $Rh_O$ (D) type |
| Antibody identification | Antibody titer | |
| | Direct Coombs test | |

(continued)

**TABLE 1-1.** *Continued*

**Clinical Immunology/Serology Procedures:**

| | | |
|---|---|---|
| Amebiasis screen | Cold agglutinins | Rheumatoid factor |
| Antinuclear AB (ANA) | CSF/VDRL | RPR |
| ASO screen | Infectious mononucleosis | RPR quantitative |
| ASO titer | MHA-TP | Salmonella agglutinins |
| Brucella abortus | Proteus OX agglutinins | Tularemia agglutinins |
| C-reactive protein | Rubella HIA | |

philia are performed in the coagulation area. Also, other procedures, such as platelet counts and fibrinogen assays, help to detect coagulation problems such as disseminated intravascular coagulation disease (DIC).

The clinical microscopy and urinalysis area utilizes microscopic and chemical procedures to screen urine specimens for abnormalities. Generally, each patient admitted to a health-care facility must have a urinalysis performed on his or her random sample (see Chapter 3 for urine collection information). Assays performed on a urine specimen include the determination of pH, specific gravity, protein, sugar, ketones, bilirubin, nitrates, urobilinogen, ascorbic acid, and occult blood. Also, a microscopic examination is performed to identify the presence or absence of crystals, casts, white blood cells, and red blood cells.

*Clinical Microbiology.* The section of clinical microbiology has the principal tasks of culturing and identifying bacterial pathogens and their toxins. In addition, this section evaluates bacterial sensitivity to a particular antibi-

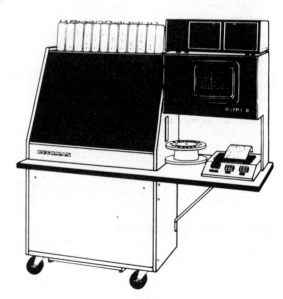

**Figure 1-7.** Photograph of ASTRA 8. *(Courtesy of Beckman Instruments, Brea, California.)*

otic. Thus, when a microbiologic specimen is collected, the physician usually requests a culture and sensitivity test (C and S). Sensitivity refers to the inhibition of bacterial growth by an antibiotic.

The bacterial pathogens are classified according to (1) how they appear after Gram staining; (2) shape of the microorganisms—rod-shaped (bacilli), circular-shaped (cocci), or spiral-shaped (spirochetes); and (3) the microorganism requirements for oxygen (aerobic) or lack of oxygen (anaerobic).

Major methods for analysis in this section include: (1) how these microorganisms grow in culture, (2) their biochemical properties, and (3) sensitivity of the microorganisms to antibiotics. In addition to analysis of bacterial pathogens, this section identifies pathogenic parasites, fungi, and viruses.

The occult (hidden) blood test (Guaiac test) is frequently performed in the clinical microbiology section. This procedure tests for blood in feces (stool), urine, and other patient's secretions.

The specimens for microbiologic analysis may be highly infectious, and thus, are considered biohazardous. Extreme caution and care must be taken in collecting and processing them.

*Clinical Immunology—Serology.* The serology section has the major tasks of running procedures to determine antigen−antibody reactions and identify

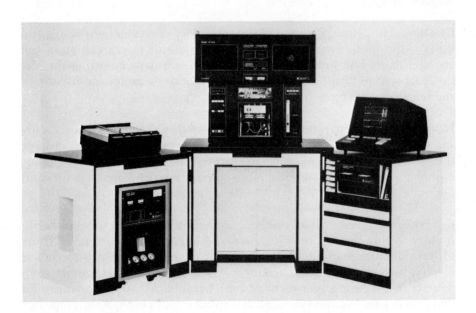

**Figure 1-8.** Photograph of Coulter Counter. *(Courtesy of Coulter Electronics, Inc., Hialeah, Florida.)*

diseases having antigen–antibody pathogenesis. Common serologic tests run in the serology–clinical immunology section include: VDRL, RPR, FTA-ABS, cold agglutinins, febrile agglutinins, rubella, ASO titer, anti-DNase B, fungus antibody tests, and Monospot. As an example of diseases that are identified in this section, the VDRL (Venereal Disease Research Laboratory) and RPR (Rapid Plasma Reagin) tests are used to test for syphilis. FTA-ABS (fluorescent treponemal antibody absorption test) is a procedure used to confirm a syphilitic infection with the spiral-shaped bacteria. The cold agglutinins test is primarily for primary atypical pneumonia. Febrile agglutinins is a procedure used to test for typhoid fever, paratyphoid, brucellosis, and tularemia. The ASO titer is used to test for a streptococci infection and Monospot (Ortho Diagnostics) tests for infectious mononucleosis.

**Blood Banking (Immunohematology).** The blood bank, sometimes referred to as immunohematology, has the major tasks of providing blood products to patients. These products collected from volunteer donors and given to the patients (recipients) include whole blood, packed red blood cells, platelets, and fresh frozen plasma. In order to give blood to patients, the donor and recipient must have their blood grouped and typed. In addition, other procedures run in the blood bank include: antibody screening test, Rh antibody titer test, direct antiglobulin (Coombs) test, and hepatitis B surface antigen ($HB_sAg$).

**Cytology.** The cytology section of the laboratory processes body fluids and other tissue specimens for detection and diagnostic interpretation of cell changes that might indicate cancer. Cytology is usually known as the section that screens "Pap" smears for early diagnosis of malignant diseases of the female genital tract.

**Histology.** The preparation and processing of tissue samples removed during surgery, autopsy, or other medical procedures are the primary tasks of the histology section. Following preparation of the tissue, the anatomic pathologist microscopically examines and evaluates the patient's tissue sample.

**Cytogenetics.** The section of cytogenetics is relatively new in the clinical laboratory. Within this section, cytogenetics techniques provide detailed study of individual chromosomes (Fig. 1-9) that detect relationships to clinical disease, both congenital and acquired. The cytogenetic tasks require competence in preparing specimens of peripheral blood, bone marrow, solid tissue, and amniotic fluid through cell cultures and chromosomal analysis. The phlebotomist, on occasions, may draw blood specimens for chromosomal analysis.

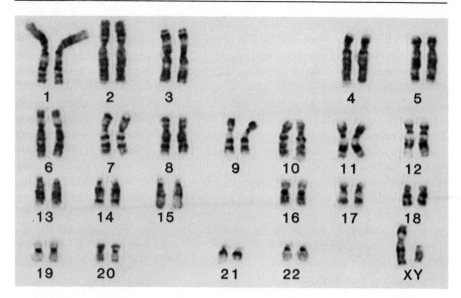

**Figure 1-9.** Photograph of karyotype. *(Courtesy of University of Texas M. D. Anderson Hospital, Department of Laboratory Medicine.)*

*Education and Research.* The large clinical laboratory usually has ongoing research in the development of new procedures recently described in the medical literature, as well as basic research contributing to the clinical laboratory sciences. This work is performed by the pathologists, other doctorate staff, and the medical technologists.

In addition to research, the large clinical laboratory department generally provides or is affiliated with a university for teaching programs. The educational programs include: (1) a pathology residency program to teach physicians the subspecialty of pathology; (2) a medical technology program to teach qualified college seniors or graduates the concepts, theories, and techniques in clinical laboratory sciences; (3) a medical laboratory technician program to train college freshmen and sophomores the basic techniques and concepts in clinical laboratory sciences; and (4) a phlebotomy program to train individuals on how to collect blood.

*Interdepartmental Relationships.* Clinical laboratory test results provide important data to the physician in diagnosing and monitoring patients and depend on smooth interrelationships with all other hospital departments. For example, a physician requests laboratory tests to be performed on a patient. The laboratory tests are performed on admission of the patient to the hospital. When the patient's specimens and the requisition slips specifying the clinical laboratory procedures to be performed arrive at the clinical laboratory, they are sent to the appropriate section(s) for analysis. The test results are recorded in the clinical laboratory and returned to the patient's medical chart to be reviewed by the attending physician. This information must be as timely as possible, and coordination between the clinical laboratory and nursing staff is important. The appropriate charges for the laboratory tests are directed to the patient's account at the business office.

Information resulting from the laboratory test requires that clinical laboratory coordinate its activities with other hospital departments such as nursing, pharmacy, and dietary. Because the effects of diet and medication(s) on laboratory test results have been well-documented, coordination and cooperation between the laboratory, medical staff, nursing staff, dietary department, and the pharmacy are required to prevent false test results. This team of health-care providers must be aware of the total patient care plan in relation to the clinical laboratory collection and test procedures so that laboratory test results can be efficiently utilized for the best possible patient care.

## STUDY QUESTIONS

1. Which of the following hospital departments uses ionizing radiation for treating diseases and fluoroscopic and radiographic x-ray instrumentation for the diagnosis of diseases?

    **a.** radiology            **c.** nuclear medicine

    **b.** radiation therapy    **d.** occupational therapy

2. The electroencephalograph (EEG) is an instrument that records:

    **a.** the electric current produced by the contraction of the heart muscle

    **b.** brain waves

    **c.** signals from the skeletal muscles

3. Which of the following clinical laboratory sections performs the VDRL?

    **a.** clinical chemistry    **c.** clinical immunology

    **b.** hematology            **d.** clinical microbiology

4. Blood glucose determinations are usually performed in which of the following laboratory sections?

    **a.** clinical chemistry    **c.** clinical immunology

    **b.** hematology            **d.** clinical microbiology

5. From the following personnel, which individual is sometimes referred to as clinical laboratory scientist?

    **a.** medical laboratory    **b.** medical technologist
        technician
                                 **c.** phlebotomist

# REFERENCES

1. Price G: American Society for Medical Technology's alternative proposal (ASMT's comments on the notice of proposed regulations on clinical laboratory personnel standards). Am J Med Technol 46:2, 1980.
2. Becan-McBride K: Textbook of Clinical Laboratory Supervision. New York, Appleton-Century-Crofts, 1982.
3. Hermann Hospital, Department of Pathology and Laboratory Medicine Personnel Policies. Houston, 1982.

# CHAPTER 2

# Anatomy and Physiology of Body Systems

Diana Garza

## ANATOMIC REGIONS

The human body has distinctive characteristics, i.e., a back bone, bisymmetry, body cavities, and nine major organ systems: skeletal, muscular, nervous, respiratory, digestive, urinary, reproductive, endocrine, and circulatory. This chapter highlights each system and emphasizes the role of the circulatory system. The front, anterior, or ventral surface of the body is separated into thoracic, abdominal, and pelvic cavities. The back, posterior, or dorsal surface is divided into cranial and spinal cavities. Each of these cavities houses one or more organs. Areas of the body can be described by their distance from or proximity to one of the body planes (Fig. 2-1). The sagittal plane runs lengthwise from front to back, dividing the body into right and left halves. The frontal plane runs lengthwise from side to side, dividing the body into anterior and posterior sections. The transverse plane runs crosswise or horizontally, dividing the body into upper and lower sections. Normal anatomic position refers to an erect standing position with arms at rest and palms forward.[1]

## MAJOR BODY FUNCTIONS

Survival is the primary function of the human body and many complex processes work independently and together to achieve this function. In human physiology, the body strives for a steady state of homeostasis. Liter-

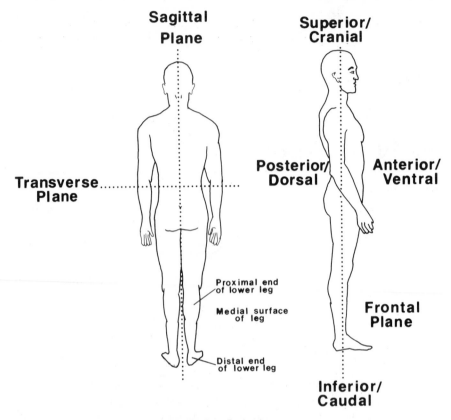

**Sagittal Plane**

**Superior/ Cranial**

**Transverse Plane**

**Posterior/ Dorsal**

**Anterior/ Ventral**

Proximal end of lower leg

Medial surface of leg

**Frontal Plane**

Distal end of lower leg

**Inferior/ Caudal**

**Figure 2-1.** Body planes.

ally, homeostasis means "remaining the same." It is a condition in which a healthy body, although constantly changing and functioning, remains in a normal healthy condition. Homeostasis, or a steady state condition, allows the normal body to keep in balance by compensating with changes. For example, if the body is taking in too much water, it responds to this imbalance by excreting water from the kidneys (urine), skin (perspiration), intestines (feces), and lungs (water in expiration) (Fig. 2-2). A healthy body maintains constancy of its chemical components and processes in order to survive. All organ systems and body structures play a part in maintaining homeostasis.

Another important function of the human body is metabolism. This is the process of making necessary substances or breaking down chemical substances in order to utilize energy. Catabolism is a series of chemical reactions produced in cells to change complex substances into simpler ones

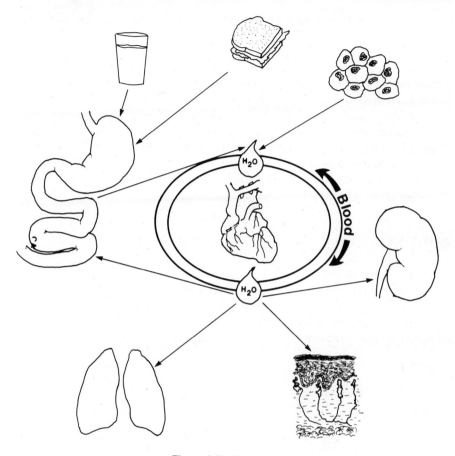

**Figure 2-2.** Homeostasis.

while simultaneously releasing energy. It provides energy for all functions of the body, whether by moving a chair or allowing a heart to beat. Anabolism is a process by which cells utilize energy to make complex compounds from simpler ones. It allows for the synthesis of body fluids such as sweat, tears, saliva, and/or chemical constituents (enzymes, hormones, and antibodies). Both phases are required to maintain metabolic functions in a healthy individual.

A normal healthy body integrates both structural and functional aspects of anatomy and physiology. Organization of all the body structures such as cells, tissues, organs, and systems, together with proper functioning such as digestion, respiration, circulation, nerve sensitivity, movement, and secretion provide for a healthy individual. Systems working together can keep a body metabolizing properly and in homeostasis, which is the basis of survival.

Laboratory testing can provide a wealth of information about the individual organ systems and the integrated processes. Specimens, such as blood, bone marrow, urine, cerebrospinal fluid, pleural fluid, biopsy tissue, seminal fluid, and others can be microscopically analyzed, assayed, and cultured to determine pathogenesis. This chapter summarizes the function of the nine organ systems (skeletal, muscular, nervous, respiratory, digestive, urinary, reproductive, endocrine, and circulatory) with emphasis on the circulatory system. Figure 2-3 depicts the variety of cells from some of the body systems.[1, 2]

## BODY SYSTEMS

### Skeletal System

The skeletal system refers to all bones and joints of the body. This system is comprised primarily of two types of tissue: bone and cartilage. Bone is composed of cells surrounded by calcified intercellular substances which allow for a rigid structure. Cartilage is composed of similar cells but these

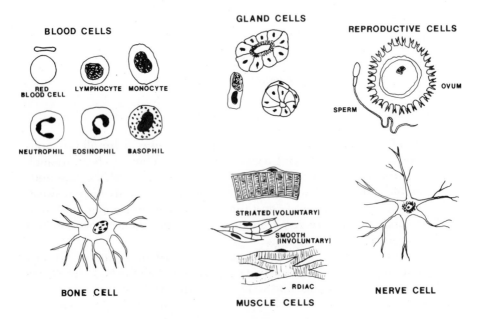

**Figure 2-3.** Various cell structures.

are surrounded by a gelatinous material instead of calcified substances, thus allowing for more flexibility. The skeletal system serves the body in five major ways: support, protection for softer tissues (brain or lungs), movement and leverage, hemopoiesis (blood cell formation) in the bone marrow, and calcium storage.

There are over 200 bones in the human body, classified into four groups based on their shapes. Long bones include leg bones, i.e., femur, tibia, fibula, and arm and hand bones, i.e., humerus, radius, ulna, and phalanges. Short bones include carpals and tarsals or wrist and ankle bones, respectively. Flat bones include several cranial bones, ribs, and scapulae or shoulder blades. And irregular bones include cranial bones, i.e., sphenoid and ethnoid, and bones of the vertebral column, i.e., vertebrae, sacrum, and coccyx (Fig. 2-4).

Bones are connected to each other by a variety of joints which permit flexion, extension, abduction (away from median), adduction (toward median), rotation, and combinations of these.

Bone structure differs between male and female skeletons. Aside from being somewhat larger and heavier, men have a pelvis that is deeper with a narrow pubic arch. The female pelvis is shallow, broad and with a wider pubic arch, to facilitate childbirth.

Laboratory assessment of the skeletal system can include serum calcium and phosphate levels, serum alkaline phosphatase (ALP) levels, microscopic analysis, and/or microbial culture of the bone marrow and/or synovial fluid (fluid between joints and bones).

## Muscular System

The muscular system refers to all muscles of the body, including those attached to bones and those along walls of internal structures such as the heart. Based on location, microscopic structure, and nervous control, muscles are classified as follows: (1) skeletal or striated voluntary—attached to bones; (2) visceral or nonstriated (smooth) involuntary—line the walls of internal structures such as veins and arteries; (3) cardiac or striated involuntary—make up the wall of the heart (Fig. 2-3). Muscles provide movement, maintain posture, and produce heat. Movement takes place not only during locomotion, but also during body movements, changes in size of openings, and propulsion of substances, i.e., blood through veins or passage of food through intestines. Posture is maintained during sitting and standing by continued partial contraction of specific muscles. Muscle cells which provide mechanical energy for movement also release energy in the form of heat. All three types of muscles work by extending, contracting, conducting, and being easily stimulated.

Laboratory testing of the muscular system often involves clinical assays of specific muscle enzymes, such as creatine kinase (CK), microscopic examination, or culturing of biopsy tissue.

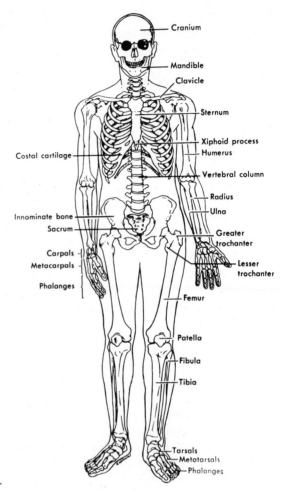

Cranium

Mandible

Clavicle

Sternum

Xiphoid process
Humerus

Costal cartilage

Vertebral column

Radius

Ulna

Innominate bone

Sacrum

Greater
trochanter

Carpals

Metacarpals

Lesser
trochanter

Phalanges

Femur

Patella

Fibula

Tibia

Tarsals
Metatarsals
Phalanges

**Figure 2-4.** The skeletal system.

## Nervous System

The nervous system provides communication in the body. Nerve impulses
and chemical substances serve to regulate, control, integrate, and organize
body functions. The nervous system is composed of specialized nerve cells
(neurons), brain, spinal cord, brain and cord coverings, fluid, and the
nerve impulse itself. Sensory neurons transmit nerve impulses to the spinal
cord or brain from muscle tissues. Motor neurons transmit impulses to
muscles from the spinal cord or brain. Both the brain and spinal cord are
covered by protective membranes (meninges). Between these protective
membrane layers are spaces filled with cerebrospinal fluid which provide a

cushion for the brain and spinal cord. The brain has many vitally important areas. In conjunction with the cranial nerves, its functions include all mental processes and many essential motor, sensory, and visceral responses. The spinal cord and spinal nerves control sensory (touch), motor (voluntary movement), and reflex (knee jerk) functions. Specific cranial and spinal nerves exist to control all complex or simple action processes in the body.

Laboratory diagnosis of nervous disorders is not very specific. Chemical assays can reveal drug interactions, as well as hormonal, protein, and enzyme alterations. Meningitis can be detected by bacterial, viral, or fungal culture or by detection of specific antibodies.

## Respiratory System

Respiration allows for the exchange of gases between blood and air. Once gases enter the blood, the circulatory system transports them between lungs and tissues. Together, the respiratory and circulatory systems get oxygen ($O_2$) to the cells and remove carbon dioxide ($CO_2$) from tissue cells. The main components of the respiratory system are housed in the head, neck, and thoracic cavity and include the nose, pharynx, larynx, trachea, bronchi, and lungs.

Receptors in the nose provide the sense of smell and allow for changes in voice. The nose also functions as the primary filter for air entering the body. It catches impurities and chemical substances that may be irritating to the respiratory system. The pharynx is a tubelike structure which allows for both food and air to pass before reaching the appropriate pathway. Along with the larynx (voice box), it determines the quality of voice. The trachea and bronchial passages provide openings for outside air to reach the lungs. Within the bronchi are grapelike alveolar sacs which are enveloped by capillaries and allow for diffusion between air and blood. The lungs are structured into millions of branches of alveoli with surrounding capillaries. They can quickly take in large amounts of oxygen ($O_2$) and release amounts of carbon dioxide ($CO_2$) if they are functioning properly. In patients with pneumonia, the alveolar sacs become inflamed and fluid or waste products block the minute air spaces, thus making normal $O_2$ and $CO_2$ exchange very difficult.

Blood transports $O_2$ and $CO_2$ as part of molecules of certain chemical compounds such as hemoglobin. When $O_2$ and $CO_2$ are exposed to blood, they rapidly combine with hemoglobin to form oxyhemoglobin and carbaminohemoglobin, respectively (Fig. 2-5).

Association and dissociation with hemoglobin depends on the gaseous pressure. In lung capillaries, $O_2$ pressure ($PO_2$) increases and $CO_2$ pressure ($PCO_2$) decreases, allowing $O_2$ to rapidly associate with hemoglobin and $CO_2$ to dissociate from carbaminohemoglobin. In tissue capillaries, the opposite occurs, $O_2$ pressure is decreased and $CO_2$ pressure increased, therefore

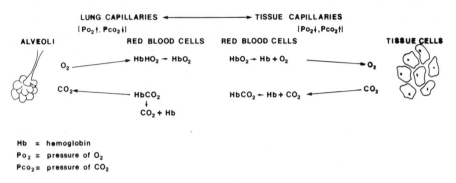

Figure 2-5. $O_2$ and $CO_2$ transport via hemoglobin.

allowing $O_2$ to dissociate from oxyhemoglobin and $CO_2$ to combine with hemoglobin.

Gas pressure can be measured in the clinical laboratory from appropriate blood samples (see Chapters 3 and 5). In addition, other tests for chemical constituents (sodium, chloride, bicarbonate, and potassium) in the blood often indicate respiratory abnormalities. Lung biopsies, throat swabs, and bronchial washings can be examined microscopically or cultured for pathogenic microorganisms such as fungi, bacteria, and acid-fast bacilli. Pathogenic microorganisms can cause infections such as tuberculosis, Legionnaire's disease, and pneumonia.

## Digestive System

The digestive system functions, first, to break down food chemically and physically into a form that can be absorbed and utilized by body cells, and second, to eliminate the waste products of digestion. The gastrointestinal (GI) tract is made up of the following components: mouth, pharynx, esophagus, stomach, intestines, and some vital accessory organs such as salivary glands, teeth, liver, gallbladder, pancreas, and appendix. Many proteins, enzymes, and juices are released by these components to facilitate digestion, absorption, and movement through the GI tract. For example, the liver secretes bile which aids in fat digestion and absorption. In addition, it is involved in carbohydrate metabolism, protein and fat catabolism, and synthesis of many vital blood proteins for clotting and regulating functions. Each component functions either mechanically or chemically to keep the body in homeostasis. The digestive system helps regulate the intake and output of essential proteins, carbohydrates, fats, minerals, vitamins, and water. The body can then utilize these substances by catabolizing them for stored energy, or anabolizing them to build other complex compounds such as hormones, other tissue proteins, and enzymes. Levels of these constituents can be clinically measured in the laboratory from blood specimens and other body fluids.

## Urinary System

The urinary system serves primarily to produce and eliminate urine. It consists of two kidneys and ureters, one bladder, and one urethra.

The kidney's main function is to regulate the amount of water, electrolytes, (sodium, potassium, chloride), and nitrogenous waste products (urea) from protein metabolism. The concentration of these blood constituents is abnormal if the kidneys are not functioning properly. As blood passes through the specialized kidney cells called glomeruli, water and solutes are filtered out. Only the necessary amounts of these substances are reabsorbed into the blood. The rest are excreted as waste products in the urine. Ureters collect urine as it is formed and transport it to the bladder. The bladder serves as a reservoir until it can be voided. The urethra is the terminal component of the urinary system. In women, it is merely a passageway from the bladder. In men, it eliminates both urine and semen from the body.

Laboratory assessment of urinary function includes detection of chemical constituents, blood, microorganisms, and cells in the urine, as well as chemical analysis of the blood. A variety of urine collection techniques and preservatives are available.

## Reproductive System

Male reproductive structures include testes, seminal vesicles, prostate, epididymis, seminal ducts, urethra, scrotum, penis, and spermatic cords. Primary functions of this system are spermatogenesis (sperm production), storage, maintenance and excretion of seminal fluid, and secretion of hormones. Female reproductive structures include ovaries, fallopian tubes, uterus, vagina, and vulva. These structures play a role in ovulation, fertilization, menstruation, pregnancy, labor, and secretion of hormones.

Laboratory tests of these reproductive functions might include semen, hormonal analysis, and cytogenic analysis, as well as microbiologic cultures of infected areas.

## Endocrine System

Endocrine glands release their secretions (hormones) directly into the bloodstream. This glandular system has the same functions as the nervous system, i.e., communication, control, and integration. Hormones play an important role in metabolic regulation that influences growth and development, in fluid and electrolyte balance, energy balance, and acid-base balance. Hormonal imbalances can lead to severe disorders such as dwarfism, giantism, and sterility. Endocrine glands include pituitary, thyroid, parathyroid, adrenal, ovaries, and testes.

Because hormones are transported via the bloodstream, it is easy to detect abnormalities by analyzing blood samples. Chemical assays are available for all types of hormones and provide very specific and sensitive patient results.

## Circulatory System

The circulatory system transports water, electrolytes, hormones, enzymes, antibodies, cells, gases, and food to all cells. In addition, it contributes to body defenses and the coagulation process. This discussion centers around the processes by which these functions occur, composition of blood, and formation of blood.

The lymphatic system is often considered to be part of the circulatory system. Its main purpose is to circulate lymph fluid to and from the tissues and to produce blood cells. Lymph tissue is found in nodes, thymus, spleen, bone marrow, liver, and tonsils.

***Blood.*** Blood is composed of water, solutes, and cells. Normally, a man has approximately 5 quarts (4.75 liters) of blood. It is composed of approximately 3 quarts of plasma and 2 quarts of cells. Plasma contains water and solutes. Cells are classified as red blood cells (RBCs or erythrocytes), white blood cells (WBCs or leukocytes), and platelets (thrombocytes). White blood cells are divided further into granulocytes (basophils, neutrophils, eosinophils), lymphocytes, and monocytes (Figs. 2-6 and 2-7).

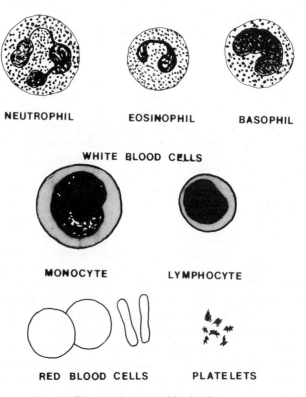

Figure 2-6. Human blood cells.

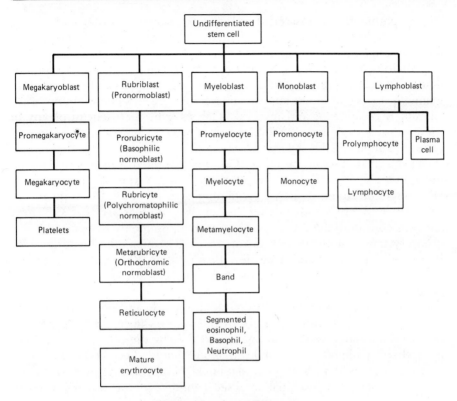

**Figure 2-7.** Blood cell formation.

*Erythrocytes.* Red blood cells measure about 7 microns in diameter. Normally, when in the circulating blood, RBCs have no nucleus. Prior to reaching maturity in the bone marrow, RBCs lose their nucleus and simultaneously become biconcaved disks. Within each mature RBC there are millions of hemoglobin molecules; each molecule is capable of carrying four oxygen molecules. As previously mentioned, hemoglobin can also carry $CO_2$.

Red blood cells are formed in the bone marrow from nucleated stem cells. Once the stem cell becomes committed to being a RBC, it matures through several stages, all of which are morphologically different. The process takes several days and the stages are called rubriblast, prorubricyte, rubricyte, metarubricyte, reticulocyte, and mature RBC. Nomenclature differs between laboratories. The terms, pronormoblast, basophilic normoblast, polychromatophilic normoblast, orthochromic normoblast are also used as indicated in Figure 2-7. The life span of RBCs is approximately 120 days in the circulating bloodstream. After this time, they begin to fragment and rupture. Cells in the liver, spleen, and bone marrow phagocytize the destroyed RBCs and begin to breakdown hemoglobin into iron-containing pigments (hemosiderin) and bile pigments (bilirubin and biliverdin). The bone marrow reuses the iron for new RBCs and the liver excretes bile pigments into the intestines.

Millions of RBCs are continually being formed and destroyed daily. The bone marrow must have an adequate supply of several substances to maintain a normal blood supply. These substances include amino acids, vitamin B complexes, and minerals such as iron. Deficiencies of any of these substances or failure of the bone marrow to function properly may result in anemia (Table 2-1).

The surface membranes of RBCs contain antigens which designate the individual's blood type. RBCs with "A" antigen are type A; those cells with "B" antigen are type B; RBCs containing both "A" and "B" antigens are type AB; and RBCs with neither "A" or "B" antigens are type O. These antigens constitute the ABO system. Another commonly recognized blood group system contains the Rh factor. If the RBCs contain the antigen for Rh factor, the individual is considered Rh positive. Rh negative people do not have the Rh factor antigen on their RBCs. Many other blood group systems exist as well.

It is vitally important that blood transfused into a patient never contain *antibodies* to the patient's blood group *antigens* on the red cells. Antibodies can react with specific RBC antigens and destroy the red cells. This happens when a patient is transfused with blood that has been accidentally mistyped or confused with another patient's. It can be rapidly fatal to the inappropriately transfused patient. (See Table 2-2 for antibodies present in various blood types.)

**TABLE 2-1. SUMMARY OF BLOOD CELLS**

| Cells | Number/Size | Function | Formation | Destruction |
|---|---|---|---|---|
| Erythrocytes (RBC) | 4.5 to 5.5 million per cu mm; size = 6 to 7 $\mu$ | Transport $O_2$ and $CO_2$ | Bone marrow | Fragmentation and removal in spleen, liver, and bone marrow; life span $\cong$ 120 days |
| Leukocytes (WBC) | 5000 to 9000 per cu mm; size = 9 to 16 $\mu$ | Defense | Granulocytes in bone marrow; nongranular WBCs in all lymphatic tissue | Removed in spleen, liver, bone marrow; life span = 24 hours to years |
| Thrombocytes (platelets) | 250,000 to 450,000 per cu mm; size = 1 to 4 $\mu$ | Clotting | Bone marrow | Removed in spleen; life span = 9 to 12 days |

**TABLE 2-2. ABO BLOOD TYPES**

| Blood Type | Antigens on RBC | Antibodies in Serum/Plasma |
|------------|-----------------|----------------------------|
| A          | A               | Anti-B                     |
| B          | B               | Anti-A                     |
| AB         | AB              | Neither anti-A or anti-B   |
| O          | None            | Anti-A, anti-B             |

Type O RBC can be transfused into any ABO type because the RBCs do not contain "A" or "B" antigen to react with either antibodies to "A" or "B" (anti-A, anti-B) present in type A or B patients.

*Leukocytes.* The different white blood cell types differ in color, size, shape, and nuclear formation. Neutrophils, eosinophils, and basophils contain cytoplasmic granules, hence they are called granulocytes. Neutrophilic granules stain bluish with neutral dyes. Their nuclei generally have two or more lobes and are often referred to as polymorphonuclear (PMN) leukocytes. Eosinophilic granules stain orange-red with acidic dyes. Their nuclei normally have two lobes. Basophilic granules stain dark purple or black with basic dyes and their nuclei are often "S" shaped. Lymphocytes and monocytes are nongranular and have relatively large nuclei (refer to Fig. 2-6).

Leukocytes function primarily as part of the body's defense mechanism. The cells phagocytize or ingest pathogenic microorganisms. Lymphocytes play a role in immunity and in production of antibodies (refer to Table 2-1).

White blood cells are formed in bone marrow and lymphatic tissues. The exact life span varies with cell type from days up to several years. Normally, blood contains 5000 to 9000 leukocytes per cu mm with designated percentages for each cell line (Table 2-3).

*Thrombocytes.* Platelets are much smaller than other blood cells. They are fragments of megakaryocytes (located in the bone) and help initiate the clotting sequence. Normally there are 250,000 to 450,000 platelets per cu mm (refer to Table 2-1).

**TABLE 2-3. WBC DIFFERENTIAL COUNT**

| Cell Line | Normal Ranges (%) | Example (%) |
|-----------|-------------------|-------------|
| Neutrophils | 65–75 | 65 |
| Basophils | 5–1 | 1 |
| Eosinophils | 2–5 | 3 |
| Monocytes | 3–8 | 6 |
| Lymphocytes | 20–25 | 25 |
| Total | 100 | 100 |

*Plasma.* The liquid portion of the blood, without cells, is called plasma. If a chemical agent or anticoagulant is added to prevent clotting, a blood sample can be separated by centrifugation into the cells and plasma (Fig. 2-8). Chapter 3 contains additional information on anticoagulants.

Plasma is composed of 90 percent water and 10 percent solutes which include nutrients such as glucose, amino acids, and fats, metabolic wastes (urea, uric acid, creatinine, and lactic acid), respiratory gases ($O_2$ and $CO_2$), regulatory substances (hormones, enzymes, and mineral salts), and protective substances (antibodies).

*Serum.* If a blood specimen is allowed to clot, the result is serum plus blood cells meshed in a fibrin clot. Serum contains essentially the same chemical constituents as plasma except that clotting factors and blood cells are contained within the fibrin clot.

**Heart.** The human heart is a muscular organ about the size of a man's closed fist. It contains four chambers and is located slightly left of the mid-

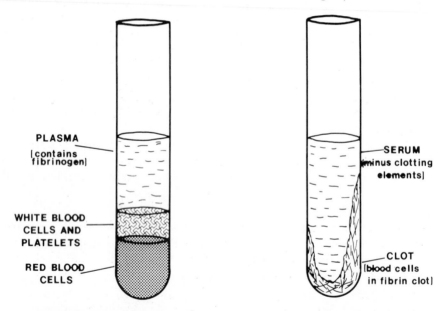

**Figure 2-8.** Blood specimens with and without anticoagulant. The blood specimen on the left is prevented from clotting by the addition of an anticoagulant and after settling or centrifugation. Plasma is approximately 90 percent $H_2O$. The remaining constituents are proteins (coagulation factors, etc.) inorganic substances (sodium, chloride, potassium etc.), organic substances (urea, creatinine, sugars, fats, cholesterol, etc.), and dissolved gases ($O_2$, $CO_2$, etc.). Red blood cells are heavier than white blood cells or platelets so they sink to the bottom. The layer of WBCs is often referred to as the "buffy coat." The blood specimen on the right will clot without anticoagulants. Serum is normally a clear, straw colored fluid which contains everything that plasma contains except the coagulation factors. A fibrin clot forms which traps RBCs, WBCs, and platelets.

line. The heart's function is to pump sufficient amounts of blood to all cells of the body by contraction (systole) and relaxation (diastole).

**Blood Vessels.** There are three kinds of blood vessels: arteries, veins, and capillaries.

*Arteries.* Vessels which carry blood away from the heart are highly oxygenated. Arteries branch into smaller vessels called arterioles. Principal arteries of the body are indicated in Figure 2-9.

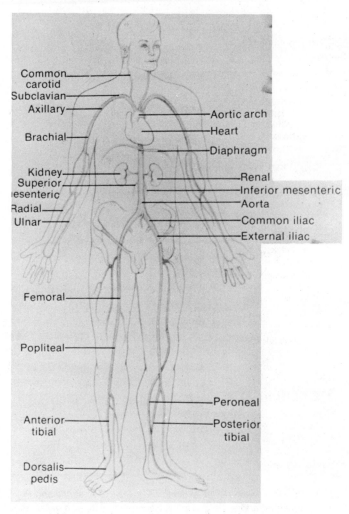

**Figure 2-9.** Principal arteries. (*From Anderson PD: Clinical Anatomy and Physiology for the Allied Health Sciences, Philadelphia, Saunders, 1976, with permission.*)

*Veins.* Blood is carried toward the heart by the smaller venules and veins. All veins except for the pulmonary veins contain deoxygenated blood. Principal veins of the body are indicated in Figure 2-10. Phlebotomists should be familiar with the principal veins of the arms and legs (Figs. 2-11 and 2-12).

*Capillaries.* Microscopic vessels which carry blood and link arterioles to venules are capillaries. Capillaries may be so small in diameter as to allow only one blood cell to pass through at any given time (Fig. 2-13).

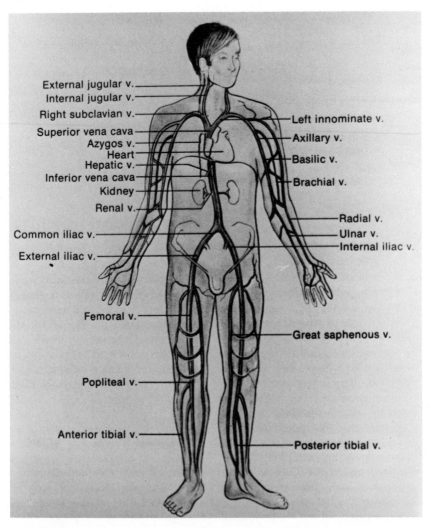

**Figure 2-10.** Principal veins. *(From Anderson PD: Clinical Anatomy and Physiology for the Allied Health Sciences, Philadelphia, Saunders, 1976, with permission.)*

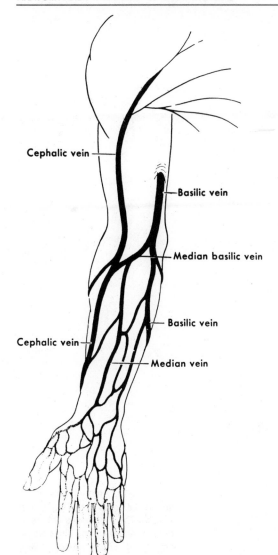

Cephalic vein

Basilic vein

Median basilic vein

Basilic vein

Cephalic vein

Median vein

**Figure 2-11.** Anterior view of the superficial veins of the arm. (*From Anthony CP, Thibodeau GA: Textbook of Anatomy and Physiology, ed 11, St. Louis, Mosby, 1983, with permission.*)

## HEMOSTASIS AND COAGULATION

Hemostasis (not to be confused with homeostasis) is concerned with the maintenance of circulating blood in the liquid state and helps retain blood in the vascular system. When there is injury to a small blood vessel, the hemostatic process serves to repair the break and arrest the hemorrhage. The first step in this process is vasoconstriction, which decreases the blood flow to the injured vessel and the surrounding vascular bed. Platelets then

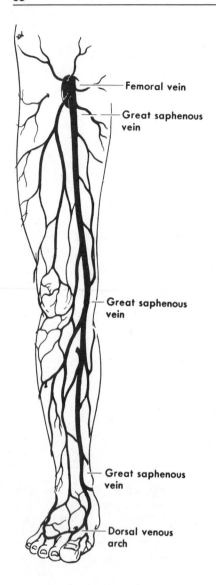

**Figure 2-12.** Anterior view of the superficial veins of the leg. (*From Anthony CP, Thibodeau GA: Textbook of Anatomy and Physiology, ed 11, St. Louis, Mosby, 1983, with permission.*)

degranulate, clump together, and adhere to the injured vessel in order to form a plug and inhibit bleeding. Many specific coagulation factors are released and interact to eventually form a fibrin meshwork or clot. Once bleeding has stopped, final repair and regeneration of the injured vessel takes place, and the clot slowly begins to degenerate.

The coagulation process is due to numerous coagulation factors. For purpose of simplicity, it is divided into two systems, intrinsic and extrinsic

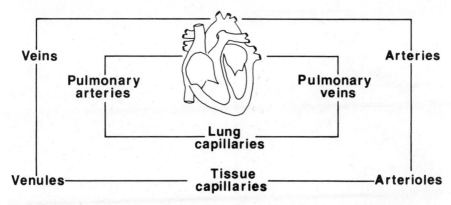

**Figure 2-13.** Schematic representation of blood pathway. $O_2$ and $CO_2$ exchange occurs in both the pulmonary and tissue capillaries.

systems. All coagulation factors required for the intrinsic system are contained in the blood. The extrinsic factors are stimulated when tissue damage occurs. Blood vessels are lined with a single layer of flat endothelial cells and are supported by subendothelial cells and collagen fibers. Normally, endothelial cells do not react or attract platelets, however, they produce and store some clotting factors. When the clotting sequence is initiated by vessel injury, they react with degranulated platelets in forming the fibrin plug (Fig. 2-14).

Large- or medium-sized veins and arteries require rapid surgical intervention to prevent bleeding. However, small arteries and veins are able to control bleeding by means of the platelet/fibrin plug and simultaneous vasoconstriction.

## LABORATORY ASSESSMENT OF THE CIRCULATORY SYSTEM

The number of RBCs, their morphology, and hemoglobin content can be measured from an anticoagulated blood specimen in the clinical hematology laboratory. Platelets and WBCs can be assessed on the basis of number and morphology. Table 2-3 illustrates the results of a laboratory procedure known as a WBC differential count whereby the specific cell lines are enumerated in percentages. Platelet function, as well as each coagulation factor can be measured from anticoagulated blood specimens in the coagulation section of the clinical hematology laboratory. Bone marrow can also be assessed in the hematology laboratory. It is removed by a physician from the sternum or iliac crest of the hip, stained, and studied microscopically for the detection of abnormal numbers and morphology of blood cells.

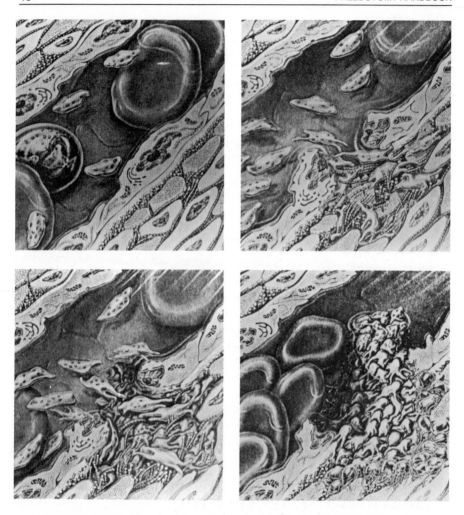

**Figure 2-14.** Sequence of hemostatic plug formation. The first sketch depicts a normal vessel. Second, a break in the vessel wall occurs and the clotting process is initiated. Third, the platelets are degranulated. Finally, the platelets and fibrin plug control bleeding. (*From Akkerman WN, et al.: Hemostasis, Boehringer Ingelheim International, 1981, with permission.*)

Tests for blood types and crossmatches for donor blood are done in an immunohematology or blood banking laboratory.

Serum and plasma constituents including nutrients, metabolic wastes, respiratory gases, regulatory substances, and protective substances can all be evaluated in the clinical chemistry laboratory. For further information on laboratory testing, see Chapter 3.

## STUDY QUESTIONS

**1.** Name the source(s) of water entry into the blood stream.

    **a.** tissue metabolism    **c.** kidneys

    **b.** food    **d.** skin

**2.** Laboratory assessment of the endocrine system routinely includes which of the following?

    **a.** blood cell analysis    **c.** lymph tissue analysis

    **b.** biopsy    **d.** hormonal analysis

**3.** Normal lung capillaries have which of the following conditions?

    **a.** increased $PO_2$    **c.** increased $PCO_2$

    **b.** decreased $PO_2$    **d.** decreased $PCO_2$

**4.** Leukocytes are formed primarily in which organs?

    **a.** central nervous system    **c.** heart

    **b.** lymphatic tissue    **d.** bone marrow

**5.** What is an anticoagulated blood specimen from venipuncture called?

    **a.** serum    **c.** plasma

    **b.** capillary blood    **d.** arterial blood

## REFERENCES

1. Anthony C: Textbook of Anatomy and Physiology. St Louis, Mosby, 1967.
2. Anderson P: Laboratory Manual and Study Guide for Clinical Anatomy and Physiology for Allied Health Sciences. Philadelphia, Saunders, 1976.

# CHAPTER 3

# Collection Reagents, Supplies, and Interfering Chemical Substances

## Kathleen Becan-McBride

## TYPES OF CLINICAL LABORATORY SPECIMENS

As described in Chapter 2, blood is composed of plasma and cells (erythrocytes, leukocytes, and thrombocytes). Almost all of the cells in the blood are erythrocytes. Plasma may be separated from blood cells by centrifugation. As shown in Figure 3-1, plasma is differentiated from serum in that plasma retains the protein clotting component, fibrinogen, which is removed from serum during the clotting process. Plasma can be obtained from whole blood that has been mixed with a chemical, an anticoagulant, to prevent clotting in the collection tube. This centrifuged blood yields plasma which contains fibrinogen in addition to the major proteins, albumin and globulin. Serum is obtained from whole blood that is not mixed with any anticoagulant. This centrifuged blood yields serum which contains albumin and globulin, but no fibrinogen.

Most clinical laboratories use serum or plasma to perform various assays. Each assay may require a different type of anticoagulant. (A discussion of these anticoagulants is included in a following section of this chapter.) Because whole blood is difficult to preserve in vitro, it is not used as often as plasma or serum in laboratory assays.

For all types of blood specimens, the phlebotomist must label the specimen with the following information: patient's name, patient's admission number, room number, date, time, and initials of phlebotomist. The prop-

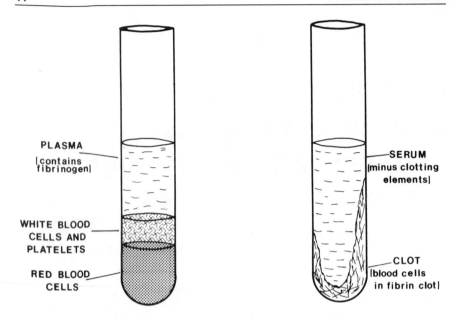

**Figure 3-1.** Differentiation between plasma and serum.

erly labeled specimens should be transported to the specimen collection area in the clinical laboratory accompanied by the laboratory request slip.

## Other Body Fluids

In addition to blood specimens, other types of body fluids are analyzed in the clinical laboratory for their various constituents. These body fluids include: (1) gastric secretions obtained by gastric intubation, (2) cerebrospinal fluid (CSF) obtained through a spinal tap or lumbar puncture, (3) synovial fluid extracted aseptically from joint cavities, and (4) fluid aspirated from body cavities (i.e., pleural fluid obtained from the lung cavity, pericardial fluid from the heart cavity, peritoneal fluid from the abdominal cavity). Phlebotomists are usually not involved in the collection of these body fluids. However, they are sometimes involved in transporting these types of specimens to the laboratory for the necessary analyses. Chemical examination, cell count, microscopic examination, and microbiologic analysis are some of the body fluid tests usually requested.

The phlebotomist should be careful in the transportation of body fluids because they are difficult to obtain and may be biohazardous. Just as for blood specimens, a laboratory request slip must accompany the body fluid specimen and the body fluid must be properly labeled (patient's name, patient's admission number, date, and time specimen collected, type of specimen, attending physician).

## Urine Collections

Because a basic urinalysis is almost always included in the routine hospital admission of a patient, the phlebotomist should be aware of the protocol for collecting the urine specimen in order to explain to the patient the proper collection technique, if such an occurrence arises.

Midstream specimens are commonly used for routine admission urinalysis. The patient is instructed to void approximately one-half of the urine into the toilet, a portion is collected in a readily available container, and the rest is allowed to pass into the toilet.[1]

If asked "what is a clean-catch urine specimen?" the phlebotomist may describe the procedure and mention that this type of specimen is used to detect the presence or absence of infecting organisms as well as routine urinalysis. The specimen must be free of contaminating matter which may be present on the external genital areas. Thus, the following steps should be explained to a female patient who is to obtain a clean-catch urine specimen:

1. The woman should separate the skin folds around the urinary opening and clean this area with a mild antiseptic soap and water;
2. Holding the skin folds apart with one hand and after urinating into the toilet, the patient should urinate into a sterile container. The container should not touch the genital area;
3. The patient should label the container with her name and time of collection and deliver to the requested place; and
4. The urine specimen should be refrigerated immediately by hospital personnel.

For a male patient, the following procedure should be adhered to for obtaining a clean-catch urine specimen:

1. The man should wash the end of his penis with soapy water and then let dry;
2. After allowing some urine to pass into the toilet, the urine should be collected in the sterile container without touching the penis; and Steps 3 and 4 are the same as for a woman.[2]

For some laboratory assays, it is necessary to analyze a 24-hour urine specimen. Incorrect collection and preservation of this type of specimen are two very frequent errors in laboratory medicine. As part of the laboratory team, the phlebotomist should be aware of the protocol for a 24-hour urine collection in order to assist other health professionals and the patient in avoiding collection errors. The following steps should be followed for a 24-hour urine collection:

1. The patient should be given a chemically clean, wide-mouthed, properly labeled container for a 24-hour urine specimen. The laboratory personnel add required preservatives to the container pri-

or to submitting it to the patient. Patients should NOT be allowed to submit urine specimens in their own jars because they may not be chemically clean and do not contain the required preservatives.

2. The patient should be instructed verbally that the collection of the 24-hour urine begins with emptying the bladder and discarding the first urine passed. This first step in the collection process should start between 6 and 8 AM with the exact time written on the container label.

3. Except for the first urine discarded, all urine should be collected during the next 24-hour period. The patient should be reminded to urinate at the end of the collection period and include this urine in the 24-hour collection.

4. Because urine is an ideal culture medium for microorganisms which decompose chemical constituents, the entire specimen should be refrigerated during collection with each specimen added during the 24-hour collection period. The patient should be told to urinate before having a bowel movement because fecal material in the urine specimen will make the specimen unacceptable for collection.

5. Some preservatives for 24-hour urine collection are very corrosive if accidentally spilled or contact is made during collection. Thus, the patient should be warned of any preservatives in the container.

6. The patient should be informed not to add anything except urine to the container and not to discard any urine during this collection period.

7. A normal intake of fluids during the collection period is desirable unless otherwise indicated by the physician.

8. Some laboratory assays require special diet restrictions, and thus, these instructions should be given to the patient.

9. If possible, medications should be discontinued for 48 to 72 hours preceding the urine collection as a precaution against interference in the laboratory assays.

10. The 24-hour urine specimen should be transported to the clinical laboratory as soon as possible. The specimen should be placed in an insulated bag or portable cooler to maintain the cool temperature.

11. Following all verbal instructions for the 24-hour urine collection, the patient should be provided with written instructions as a reminder.[3]

## Culture Specimens

Other specimens that the phlebotomist may be requested to transport to the clinical laboratory include sputum (fluid from the lungs containing pus), throat and sinus drainage cultures, wound cultures, ear or eye cultures, skin cultures, and feces. The phlebotomist should be extremely careful in the transportation of each type of specimen because they can be easily contaminated and may be biohazardous.

## INTERFERENCE OF DRUGS AND OTHER SUBSTANCES IN BLOOD

Many prescribed drugs can interfere with clinical laboratory determinations or physiologically alter the levels of blood constituents measured in the clinical laboratory. Interference of drugs and other substances is so complicated and dependent upon the chemical procedures used that only general recommendations are described here.

The direct analytical interference of drugs is decreasing with the advent of more specific and sensitive chemical procedures. However, the physiologically induced abnormalities from various types of drugs are the major causes of interference from medications. Drugs administered to alleviate an illness can induce physiologic abnormalities in one or more of the following systems: hepatic, hematologic, hemostatic, muscular, pancreatic, and renal with the resultant obscuration of the clinical diagnosis.

Prior to the laboratory measurement of chemical constituents, the attending physician should take the necessary precautions in prescribing drugs to the patient. If the patient must be maintained on medication(s) that may cause interferences in laboratory assays, the medication(s) should be written on the laboratory request form. Unless interference of medications can be avoided by ordering different laboratory assays, medications should be discontinued if at all possible, and assays repeated when false laboratory values are suspected.

Direct analytical interference in laboratory determinations is least likely to occur in blood assays because drug concentrations are usually very low. However, some drugs or drug metabolites in blood can directly cause falsely decreased or falsely elevated values in laboratory methodology.

Drug interferences leading to falsely decreased results in blood specimens may be caused by inhibition of the chromogenic or fluorescent reaction. Examples of such drugs are indicated in Table 3-1. A more complete list of such drugs can be found in Hansten's *Drug Interactions*.[4] These drugs can:

1. diminish fluorescence of the blood analyte by quenching the fluorescent energy, and thus falsely decrease the analyte's concentration;
2. compete with the blood analyte for a chromogenic reagent and thus, falsely decrease the resultant color and concentration of the analyte;
3. compete with the chromogenic reagent for peroxide in a peroxide generating reaction, and thus, falsely decrease the chromogen oxidation and concentration of the blood analyte.

**TABLE 3-1. DRUG INTERFERENCES LEADING TO FALSELY DECREASED RESULTS IN BLOOD SPECIMENS**

| Analyte | Method | Drug Interference |
|---------|--------|-------------------|
| Albumin | Colorimetric | Aspirin[4] |
| Calcium | Fluorometric | Sulfadiazine[5] |
| Glucose | Colorimetric | Ascorbic acid[6] |
| | Chromogenic oxidation (hexokinase method) | L-dopa[7] Ascorbic acid[3] |
| | Chromogenic oxidation (oxidase method) | Tetracycline[8] |
| Phosphate | Colorimetric | Phenothiazine[9] |

The falsely decreased values of the blood analyte can be mistakenly interpreted as normal or subnormal if the blood analyte was truly in an elevated range or normal range, respectively.

Drug interferences leading to falsely elevated results of blood analytes may be caused by increasing the color or fluorescence produced in the laboratory methodology and/or altering the binding characteristics in radioimmunoassays and enzyme immunoassays. Examples of such drugs are shown in Table 3-2.

Interference from medications usually causes falsely elevated values rather than falsely decreased values. Some drugs, such as acetaminophen and erythromycin, can increase serum aspartate aminotransferase and bilirubin, and thus, falsely create a clinical interpretation of hepatic dysfunction without the true presence of hepatic abnormality.[5,6] Drug-induced elevations of blood constituents can be mistakenly interpreted as falsely increased or normal whereas the true values are in the normal range or subnormal range, respectively.

Physiologically, drugs can alter blood analytes through various metabolic reactions; the production of blood cells and platelets and their survival times can be changed. Chemotherapeutic drugs can lead to a decrease in all forms of blood cellular elements and thus, their metabolic and immunologic processes.

**TABLE 3-2. DRUG INTERFERENCES LEADING TO FALSELY ELEVATED RESULTS IN BLOOD SPECIMENS**

| Analyte | Method | Drug Interference |
|---------|--------|-------------------|
| Alanine aminotransferase | Colorimetric | Erythromycin[11] |
| Bilirubin | Colorimetric | Ascorbic acid[12] Isoniazid[8] L-dopa[12] |
| Catecholamines | Fluorescent | Ampicillin[8] Ascorbic acid[8] Methyldopa[13] |
| Thyroxine | Radioimmunoassay | Oral contraceptives[3] |

**TABLE 3-3. DRUGS TOXIC TO THE LIVER[14]**

| | | |
|---|---|---|
| Salicylates | Penicillin | Acetaminophen |
| Mitomycin | Isoniazid | Chlorpromazine |
| Actinomycin | | Methyldopa |

A variety of medications (Table 3-3) are toxic to the liver and thus, can lead to acute hepatic necrosis.[14] The hepatic dysfunction, in turn, leads to an increase in blood liver enzymes such as alanine aminotransferase, alkaline phosphatase, and lactate dehydrogenase. Also, the production of globulins and clotting factors are decreased in drug-induced hepatoxicity.

Patients receiving medications that may result in renal impairment should be monitored for possible electrolyte imbalance and elevation of blood urea nitrogen. Antihypertensive agents given over a long period of time can lead to kidney damage if not monitored closely.

Pancreatitis can be caused by corticosteroids, estrogens, and diuretics[15] and causes elevations of serum amylase and lipase values.

Because many metabolic activities can be altered by medications as described in the examples above, the attending physician must note on the laboratory request form the presence of medications being taken by the patient. As a general rule, the College of American Pathologists (CAP)[16] recommends that medications that might interfere in laboratory assays be avoided for at least 4 to 24 hours prior to blood studies and 48 to 72 hours prior to urine studies. This recommendation should be followed only if no risk or serious discomfort will result in the patient.

The phlebotomist is the link between the clinical laboratory and the patient. For example, if the phlebotomist oversees the nurse administering medication(s) to the patient during the time that blood is collected for laboratory assays, the phlebotomist should communicate the patient's name and possible drug interference to the clinical laboratory supervisor in charge of specimen collection. The supervisor can then communicate with the attending physician to determine if the medication(s) will or will not interfere in the laboratory assays. The follow-up communication by the phlebotomist and clinical laboratory supervisor can lead to better patient care by avoiding interfering substances in laboratory determinations.

## SELECTION AND USE OF EQUIPMENT

Blood is the most frequent specimen analyzed in the clinical laboratory. Venipuncture with a vacuum tube (Vacutainer*), as shown in Figure 3-2, is the most direct and efficient method to obtain a blood specimen. Vacuum tubes may contain silicon to decrease the possibility of hemolysis and pre-

---

*Becton-Dickinson and Company, Rutherford, New Jersey.

vent the clot from adhering to the wall of the tube. This convenient system eliminates the need for syringes and uses disposable needles and tubes. The tubes are available in different sizes (2, 4, 5, 6, 10, 15, and 20 ml per tube) and can be purchased with different types of anticoagulants as well as chemically clean or sterile glassware. The tubes are used in conjunction with a holder-needle combination as shown in Figure 3-3. Because the needles are disposable, it eliminates the hazard of transmitting hepatitis. Each vacuum tube is color-coded according to the anticoagulant contained within the tube.

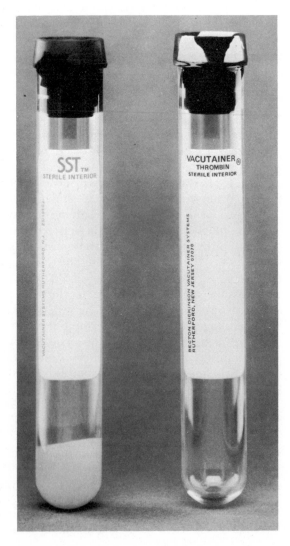

**Figure 3-2.** Vacuum tube (Vacutainer). *(Courtesy of Becton-Dickinson and Company, Rutherford, New Jersey.)*

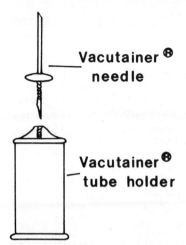

Vacutainer ®
needle

Vacutainer ®
tube holder

**Figure 3-3.** Holder-needle combination.

### Anticoagulants

Many coagulation factors are involved in blood clotting and coagulation can be prevented by the addition of different types of anticoagulants. These anticoagulants often contain preservatives that can extend the metabolism and life span of the RBCs after blood collection. Anticoagulants and preservatives are used extensively in blood donations to insure the biochemical balance of certain components of RBCs such as hemoglobin, pH, adenosine triphosphate (ATP), and glucose. Once transferred, anticoagulants, such as citrate phosphate dextrose (CPD) and acid citrate dextrose (ACD), insure that the RBCs provide the recipient with the means of delivering oxygen to the tissues.

Another major use of anticoagulants and preservatives is in the collection of plasma for laboratory analysis. Specific anticoagulants or preservatives must be used depending on the test procedure ordered. Anticoagulants cannot be substituted one for another.

Coagulation of blood can be prevented by the addition of oxalates, citrate, ethylenediaminetetraacetate (EDTA), or heparin. Oxalates, citrates, and EDTA prevent the coagulation of blood by removing calcium and forming insoluble calcium salts. Oxalates and citrates are frequently used in coagulation blood studies. EDTA prevents platelet aggregation and is therefore used for platelet counts and platelet function tests. Fresh EDTA anticoagulated blood allows for the preparation of blood films with minimal distortion of WBCs. Heparin prevents blood clotting by the inactivation of the blood clotting chemicals—thrombin and thromboplastin. Heparin is a mucopolysaccharide which is used in assays such as ammonia and plasma hemoglobin.

In addition to using the correct anticoagulant for a specific laboratory assay, the correct amount or dilution of anticoagulant in the blood speci-

TABLE 3-4. SPECIMEN TYPE AND COLLECTION TUBES

| Specimen Type | Collection Tubes (Stopper Color/Type) | Additive | Volume Draw (ml) |
|---|---|---|---|
| Blood/serum | 1) Gray and red | Inert polymer barrier | 6.0 |
| | 2) Red | None | 7.0 |
| | 3) Red | None | 2.0 |
| | 4) Red (microtainer) | Inert polymer barrier | 0.6 |
| Blood/plasma | 1) Blue | Sodium citrate | 4.5 |
| | 2) Blue | Sodium citrate | 2.7 |
| | 3) Blue | Sodium citrate | 1.8 |
| | 4) Gray | Potassium oxalate and sodium fluoride | 7.0 |
| | 5) Green | Lithium heparin | 10 |
| | 8) Royal blue or green | Sodium heparin | 10 |
| Whole blood | 1) Lavender | EDTA | 5.0 |
| | 2) Lavender | EDTA | 2.0 |

men is important. An incorrect amount of anticoagulant may lead to latent fibrin formation in the serum.

Gray stoppered Vacutainer tubes usually contain: (1) potassium oxalate and sodium fluoride or (2) sodium fluoride and thymol. This type of collection tube is used primarily for glycolytic inhibition tests. Also, some gray stoppered tubes contain only potassium oxalate and are used for laboratory assays requiring plasma or whole blood.

The anticoagulants, sodium heparin and lithium heparin, are found in green stoppered vacuum tubes. These tubes are used in various laboratory assays requiring plasma or whole blood. When used for cytogenetic studies, it is important for these tubes to be sterile.

The purple stoppered vacuum tubes (containing EDTA) are used for most hematology procedures. Many coagulation procedures are done on blood collected in blue stoppered vacuum tubes which contain sodium citrate at a concentration of 3.8 percent. Black stoppered vacuum tubes may be ordered with the following anticoagulants: (1) sodium citrate at a concentration of 3.2 percent, (2) ammonium oxalate and potassium oxalate needed for certain hematology procedures, or (3) sodium oxalate that is used to collect blood for routine coagulation procedures.

Dependent upon the needs of the laboratory procedure, the tubes may be ordered with or without sterilization. Sterile vacuum collecting tubes are frequently used in the following procedures: LE cell preparation, prothrombin time, sedimentation rate, trace element studies, and activated clotting time. Sterile blood specimens are also ordered for blood cultures when the patient is suspected of having septicemia (symptoms of sepsis). A major problem with collecting blood for culture is that the patient's sample can become contaminated with microorganisms from the skin. Thus, the blood must be collected in a sterile container (vacuum tube or syringe) under aseptic conditions.

As shown in Figure 3-4, blood can be collected directly into vacuum tubes that contain culture media. This type of collection minimizes the risk of specimen contamination. The vacuum tubes can be purchased with: (1) different types of culture media, (2) an unplugged venting unit for aerobic incubation, and/or (3) a plugged venting unit for anaerobic incubation.

Blood collecting vacuum tubes can be ordered in different sizes to allow for the different amounts of blood needed for various types of clinical laboratory assays. Table 3-5 lists the laboratory assays with the types of anticoagulants required and the approximate milliliters of blood needed to be drawn.

### Syringes and Needles

Some patients' veins are too fragile to collect blood using the vacuum tubes. Thus, syringes must be used for the collection process. Syringes, as well as tubes, must be chemically clean in order to avoid any interfering effects with the constituents to be measured. In general, syringes and tubes do not have to be sterile to measure chemical constituents. The phlebotomist should know whether the tubes or syringes to be used in collection are sterile or chemically clean because a sterile tube or syringe does not indicate that the collecting device is also chemically clean. The syringe must be the correct size for the amount of blood to be collected. Disposable plastic syringes are most frequently used. Infrequently, a glass syringe is needed to collect blood for a special procedure, and thus, the glass plunger and barrel should be inspected carefully before using.

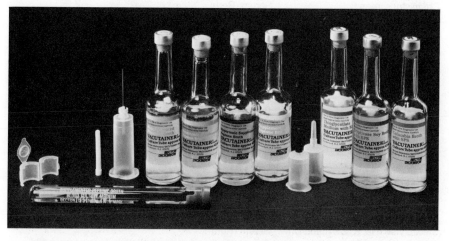

**Figure 3-4.** Vacutainer Microbiology Specimen Collection Units. *(Courtesy of Becton-Dickinson and Company, Rutherford, New Jersey.)*

## TABLE 3-5. LABORATORY ASSAYS AND THE REQUIRED TYPES OF ANTICOAGULANTS

| Test Name | Specimen Type/Stopper Color | Whole Blood Minimum Volume (ml) |
| --- | --- | --- |
| Acetaminophen | Serum (Red) | 2 |
| Acetone | Serum (Red) | 1 |
| Acid phosphatase | Serum (Red) | 2 |
| Alcohol | Serum (Red) | 3 |
| Alkaline phosphatase | Serum (Red) | 1 |
| Alpha-1-antitrypsin | Serum (Red) | 1 |
| Alpha-2-macro globulin | Serum (Red) | 1 |
| Ammonia | Plasma (Green) | 3 |
| Ampicillin | Serum (Red) | 5 |
| Amylase | Serum (Red) | 1 |
| Anticonvulsants (Dilantin, Mysoline, phenobarb, carbamazepine, valproic acid) | Serum (Red) | 7 |
| APTT | Plasma (Blue) | 1.8 |
| ASO Titer | Serum (Red) | 3 |
| Barbiturates | Serum (Red) | 2 |
| Bilirubin, total and/or direct | Serum (Red) | 1 |
| Bromide | Serum (Red) | 2 |
| Brucella | Serum (Red) | 2 |
| BSP | Serum (Red) | 3 |
| BUN | Serum (Red) | 1 |
| Calcium | Serum (Red) | 1 |
| Calcium, ionized | Serum (Red) | 2 |
| Carbamazepine (Tegretol) | Serum (Red) | 2 |
| Carbenicillin | Serum (Red) | 5 |
| Carbon dioxide | Serum (Red) | 2 |
| Carotene | Serum (Red) | 3 |
| Chemistry screen | Serum (Red) | 2 |
| Chloride | Serum (Red) | 3 |
| Cholesterol | Serum (Red) | 1 |
| Cholinesterase | Serum (Red) | 3 |
| Chloramphenicol | Serum (Red) | 5 |
| Complement ($C_3$-$C_4$) | Serum (Red) | 5 |
| CBC | Whole Blood (Purple) | 2 |
| Copper | Plasma (Blue) | 3 |
| Cortisol | Plasma (Purple) | 2 |
| CPK | Serum (Red) | 1 |
| C-reactive protein | Serum (Red) | 2 |
| Creatinine | Serum (Red) | 1 |
| Cryofibrinogen | Plasma (Green) | 1 |
| Cryoglobulin | Serum (Red) | 4 |
| Digitoxin | Serum (Red) | 2 |
| Digoxin | Serum (Red) | 2 |
| Dilantin (phenytoin) | Serum (Red) | 2 |
| Electrolytes (Na, K, $CO_2$, and Cl) | Serum (Red) | 2 |
| Electrophoresis (SPE) | Serum (Red) | 1 |
| Eosinophil count | Whole Blood (Purple) | 1 |

*(continued)*

**TABLE 3-5.** *Continued*

| Test Name | Specimen Type/Stopper Color | Whole Blood Minimum Volume (ml) |
|---|---|---|
| Erythromycin | Serum (Red) | 5 |
| ESR | Whole Blood (Purple) | 2.0 |
| Euglobulin lysis | Plasma (Blue) | 4.5 |
| Factor assays | Plasma (Blue) | 4.5 |
| Fasting blood glucose | Plasma (Gray) | 1 |
| FTA-ABS | Serum (Red) | 3 |
| Fibrinogen | Plasma (Blue) | 1.8 |
| Folate, serum | Serum (Red) | 5 |
| Fluoride | Serum (Red) | 6 |
| Folate, whole blood (RBC and serum) | Whole Blood (Purple) | 3 |
| Gamma-glutamyl transpeptidase | Serum (Red) | 1 |
| Gentamicin | Serum (Red) | 5 |
| Glucose (FBS and tolerance) | Plasma (Gray) | 1 |
| Haptoglobin | Serum (Red) | 1 |
| Hematology battery | Whole Blood (Purple) | 2 |
| IgA | Serum (Red) | 1 |
| IgD | Serum (Red) | 1 |
| IgG | Serum (Red) | 1 |
| IgM | Serum (Red) | 1 |
| Infectious mono | Serum (Red) | 1 |
| Inhibitor assay | Plasma (Blue) | 4.5 |
| Inhibitor screen | Plasma (Blue) | 4.5 |
| Insulin (on ice) | Plasma (Purple) | 3 |
| Iron profile (Iron, TIBC, and saturation) | Serum (Red) | 3 |
| Kanamycin | Serum (Red) | 5 |
| Lactate dehydrogenase (LDH) | Serum (Red) | 2 |
| Lactic acid (on ice) | Plasma (Gray) | 3 |
| Lipoprotein | Serum (Red) | 1 |
| Lithium | Serum (Red) | 2 |
| Lysozyme, serum | Serum (Red) | 2 |
| Magnesium, serum | Serum (Red) | 3 |
| Methicillin | Serum (Red) | 5 |
| Methotrexate | Serum (Red) | 2 |
| Monospot | Serum (Red) | 1 |
| Osmolality, serum | Serum (Red) | 2 |
| Penicillin | Serum (Red) | 5 |
| Phenobarbital | Serum (Red) | 2-1 |
| Phenytoin (Dilantin) | Serum (Red) | 2-1 |
| Phosphorus, serum | Serum (Red) | 2-1 |
| Plasma, Hgb | Plasma (Green) | 1 |
| Platelets | Whole Blood (Purple) | 2 |
| Potassium | Serum (Red) | 2 |
| Primidone (Mycoline) | Serum (Red) | 2 |
| Procainamide, N-acetyl-procainamide | Serum (Red) | 2 |

*(continued)*

**TABLE 3-5.** *Continued*

| Test Name | Specimen Type/Stopper Color | Whole Blood Minimum Volume (ml) |
|---|---|---|
| Prolactin | Serum (Red) | 2-1 |
| Pronestyl (Procainamide) | Serum (Red) | 2 |
| Protein, total | Serum (Red) | 1 |
| Protime | Plasma (Blue) | 1.8 |
| Proteus OX 19 | Serum (Red) | 2 |
| Quinidine | Serum (Red) | 2-1 |
| Renin activity (on ice) | Plasma (Purple) | 5 |
| Reticulocyte | Whole Blood (Purple) | 1 |
| Rheumatoid factor assay | Serum (Red) | 2 |
| Rubella | Serum (Red) | 2 |
| Salicylate | Serum (Red) | 2 |
| Salmonella | Serum (Red) | 6 |
| Sedimentation rate (ESR) | Whole Blood (Purple) | 2.0 |
| Sickling screen | Whole Blood (Purple) | 1 |
| SPE | Serum (Red) | 1 |
| SGOT (AST) | Serum (Red) | 2 |
| SGPT (ALT) | Serum (Red) | 2 |
| Sodium, serum | Serum (Red) | 2 |
| Streptozyme | Serum (Red) | 2 |
| Syphilis, standard test | Serum (Red) | 3 |
| Transferrin | Serum (Red) | 2 |
| Theophylline (Aminophyline) | Serum (Red) | 2 |
| Thrombin time | Plasma (Blue) | 4.5 |
| Triglyceride | Serum (Red) | 2 |
| Urea nitrogen | Serum (Red) | 1 |
| Uric acid | Serum (Red) | 1 |
| Valproic acid (Depakene) | Serum (Red) | 2 |
| VDRL | Serum (Red) | 3 |
| Viscosity | Serum (Red) | 3 |
| Vitamin A | Serum (Red) | 3 |
| Vitamin $B_{12}$ | Serum (Red) | 2 |
| Volatiles | Serum (Red) | 2 |
| D-xylose | Serum (Red) | 3 |

The gauge and length of a needle used on a syringe or vacuum tube is selected according to the specific task. For example, larger needles (18 gauge) are used in collecting donor units of blood (up to 450 ml), whereas smaller needles (21 and 22 gauge) are used to collect specimens for laboratory assays. The gauge number indicates the diameter of the needle, and the smaller the number, the larger the needle. The length of the needle depends upon the depth of a vein. The tip of the needle should be checked for damage; a blunt or bent tip can be harmful to the patient's vein and may lead to failure of blood collection.

After the blood is drawn by syringe, it should be immediately transferred to a chemically clean, dry tube. The needle must be removed from the syringe to avoid hemolysis before transferring the blood. The blood should be allowed to clot for a minimum of 15 minutes at room temperature, and longer if it is refrigerated. If the clot adheres to the wall of the tube, the phlebotomist or other laboratory personnel should "ring" the tube before centrifugation. "Ringing" is done by making a sweeping motion around the inside of the tube with a wooden applicator stick. However, excessive "ringing" increases the chances of hemolysis. If the clot is allowed to retract for a longer period of time, the chances for hemolysis are decreased and the yield of serum is enhanced. The longer the blood cells remain in contact with the serum, the greater the shift of substances from blood cells to serum through the metabolic process of glycolysis.

## Separation Tubes

An alternative procedure is to draw blood into a serum separation tube such as the Monoject Corvac.† Blood is collected in the vacuum Corvac tube using conventional blood collecting techniques. As illustrated in Figure 3-5, this tube contains a gel in a cup-shaped plastic "energizer" containing microscopic glass particles. As blood enters the tube, the glass particles go into suspension and accelerate clotting by providing increased surface area. As shown in Figure 3-6, when the blood in the Corvac tube is centrifuged, the energizer cup displaces the gel and forces it from the bottom to the sides of the tube. The gel's specific gravity is intermediate to serum and clotted blood. Thus, it stops moving when the equilibrium point is reached. At this point, the gel forms a positive, stable, chemical and physical barrier between the clotted blood and serum for up to 24 hours after centrifugation.

## The Butterfly

The butterfly is the most commonly used intravenous device. It is a stainless steel beveled needle and tube with attached plastic wings as shown in Figure 3-7. A variation of the butterfly is the heparin lock. The most common butterfly sizes are 19 and 21 gauge needles. The butterfly is sometimes used in the collection of blood from patients who are difficult to stick by conventional methods.

## Tourniquets

The tourniquet is a key to successful venipuncture; it provides a barrier against venous flow. Tourniquets that are used include: (1) penrose, (2) strap, (3) rubber hose, and (4) blood pressure cuff. The blood pressure cuff can be used very successfully when veins are difficult to find. The most efficient blood barrier provides a resistance that is less than systolic blood pres-

---

†Monoject Scientific, a Division of Sherwood Medical.

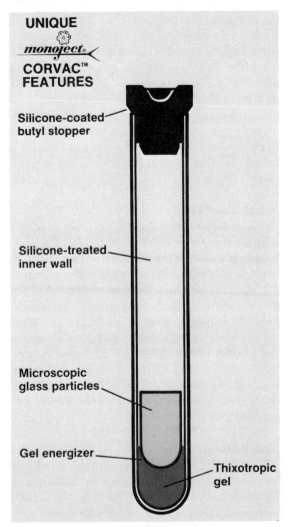

**UNIQUE**

*monoject*

**CORVAC™ FEATURES**

Silicone-coated butyl stopper

Silicone-treated inner wall

Microscopic glass particles

Gel energizer

Thixotropic gel

**Figure 3-5.** Corvac tube. *(Courtesy of Monoject Scientific, a Division of Sherwood Medical.)*

sure, but greater than diastolic; or stated another way, blood flows in, but not out. The blood pressure cuff can determine these pressures, and consequently, is a perfect tourniquet.[17]

## MICROCOLLECTION EQUIPMENT

Usually, capillary blood collecting techniques are used on infants because venipuncture is excessively hazardous. Capillary collection is indicated in adults for the following reasons: (1) severely burned, (2) veins that are difficult to stick due to their small size or location, or (3) extreme obesity.

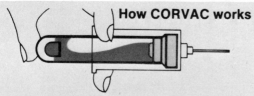

# How CORVAC works

**1.** The CORVAC tube utilizes traditional phlebotomy techniques.

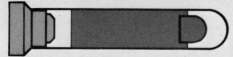

**2.** Powdered glass suspended throughout the sample accelerates coagulation.

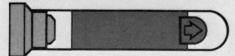

**3.** Centrifugal force drives the gel energizer into the silicone gel at the base of the tube.

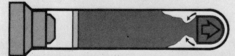

**4.** The energizer controls the flow of the gel up the sides of the tube.

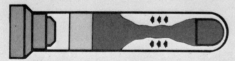

**5.** The gel continues to move up the sides of the tube, seeking an equilibrium between serum and coagulum.

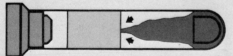

**6.** The gel reaches an equilibrium between serum and coagulum.

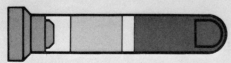

**7.** The gel forms a stable barrier between serum and coagulum.

**Figure 3-6.** How the Corvac works. *(Courtesy of Monoject Scientific, a Division of Sherwood Medical.)*

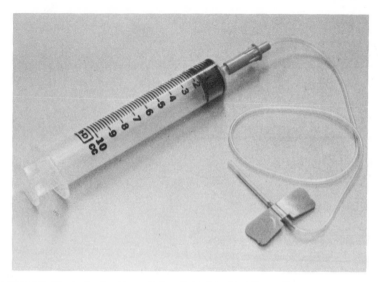

**Figure 3-7.** The butterfly. *(From Abbott Hospitals, Inc., North Chicago, Ill., and Becton-Dickinson and Company, Rutherford, New Jersey.)*

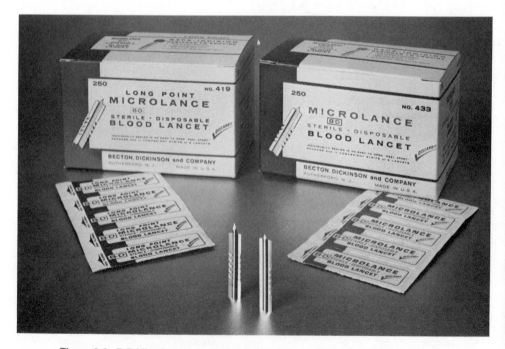

**Figure 3-8.** B-D Microlance—A single-use blood lancet. *(Courtesy of Becton-Dickinson and Company, Rutherford, New Jersey.)*

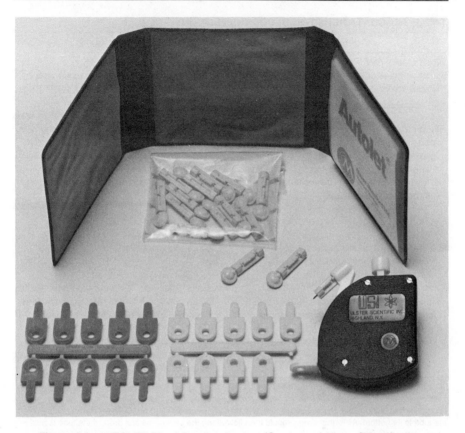

**Figure 3-9.** AUTOLET Blood Drawing Device. *(Courtesy of Ulster Scientific, Inc., (USI), Highland, New York.)*

The volume of plasma or serum that generally can be collected from a premature infant is approximately 100 to 150 $\mu$l, and about two times that amount from a full-term newborn. Larger volumes are obtained from older children and adults.[18]

A disposable sterile lancet should be used to puncture the skin for capillary collection. In newborns, lancets with tips 2.5 mm or less in length, such as the B-D Microlance (Fig. 3-8), are required to avoid penetrating bone. The Committee on Pediatric Clinical Chemistry (CPCC) favors the B-D Microlance and the Monolet lancet by Monojet.*[19] Longer tips (5 mm maximal length) are suitable for older children. Another method of micro-collection is by the AUTOLET‡ as shown in Figure 3-9. It is a spring acti-

---

*Monoject Scientific, a Division of Sherwood Medical.
‡Ulster Scientific, Inc., Highland, New York.

**TABLE 3-6. CONTAINERS FOR BLOOD COLLECTION**

| Container[a] | Remarks |
| --- | --- |
| *Blood Gases (pH, $P_{CO_2}$, $P_{O_2}$):* | |
| Natelson glass collecting pipets, 75 and 250µl volumes, ammonium heparin | To mix, insert metal "fleas" or mixing bars, after filling.[b] Seal with caps or sealing wax. Mix by use of a magnet. *Source:* Many laboratory suppliers. |
| Blood-collecting pipet kits and component parts, supplied by manufacturers of blood-gas apparatus | Kits containing glass capillaries, sealing wax, metal mixing bars, and magnets. *Source:* Laboratory suppliers of Corning, Illinois, and Radiometer equipment. |
| Caraway glass tubes, 370µl volume, ammonium heparin | Mix and seal as above, or by inversion. *Source:* Many laboratory suppliers. |
| *Electrolytes ($CO_2$, Cl, K, Na) and General Chemistry:* | |
| Microhematocrit glass capillary tubes 1.1 to 1.2 mm i.d., 75 mm long, ammonium heparin | Plasma obtained. Mix and seal as above. |
| Micro sample tubes, polyethylene, 250µl, lithium heparin; larger sizes (400-, 500-µl) for general chemistry, with and without heparin. | Plasma obtained. Seal with attached cap. Mix by inversion.[c] *Source:* Kew Scientific and Beckman Instruments, Inc. |
| B-D Microtainer, polypropylene, 600µl, silicone separator (58). | Serum obtained. Seal with accompanying cap. Centrifuge at 6000 × g. *Source:* Becton-Dickinson and Co. |

[a]Containers listed here are all commercially available.
[b]Mixing without a flea is also possible by gently inverting the capillary before sealing.
[c]For collecting electrolytes, fill two 250µl tubes, one for $CO_2$/Cl, another for Na/K. Shake the first drop entering the tube to its bottom. All further drops should then flow along the path of the first drop, if the tube is held in a nearly vertical position.
*(From Meites, S: Pediatric Clinical Chemistry, 1981.[19])*

vated puncture device with two disposable platforms for control of penetration depth. Scalpel blades that do not have appropriate control of the cutting edge and depth of puncture should not be used.

Microcontainers used by the CPCC for blood gases, electrolytes, and general chemistry collections are shown in Table 3-6. Usually, microspecimens for blood gases are collected in heparinized glass Natelson tubes. The blood collected in these tubes must be mixed with the heparin by a small metal "flea" or bar with a magnet. After mixing, the ends are sealed with sealing wax or plastic caps.

Electrolytes and general chemistry microspecimens can be collected in the B-D Microtainer† tube that has its own capillary blood collector, self-contained serum separator, and red stopper, as shown in Figure 3-10. This

†Becton-Dickinson and Company, Rutherford, New Jersey.

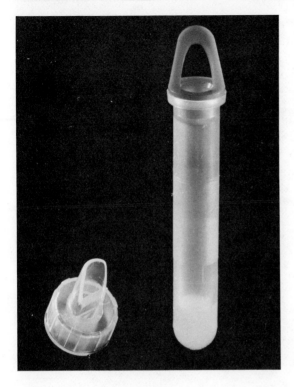

**Figure 3-10.** Microtainer tube. *(Courtesy of Becton-Dickinson and Company, Rutherford, New Jersey.)*

system can collect up to 600 μl of blood. Alternately, two or more capillary tubes can be used for electrolyte and general chemistry collection. An advantage of these tubes is that if blood is hemolyzed in one capillary tube, another capillary tube containing the patient's sample can be used for the chemical analyses.

For most chemical assays, lithium and ammonium salts of heparin are the anticoagulants of choice for microcollections. They have rarely been reported to interfere with the determination of blood gases, electrolytes, and most other chemical assays.[20]

Another type of microcollection device is the B-D Unopette† as shown in Figure 3-11. This device serves as a collection and dilution unit for blood samples, and thus increases the speed and simplicity of laboratory procedures. They are prefilled with specific amounts of diluents or reagents or both for different types of laboratory assays. Some of the more prevalent procedures in which Unopettes are used include white blood cell count, red blood cell count, platelet count, hemoglobin, RBC fragility test, sodium and potassium, and lead.

---

†Becton-Dickinson and Company, Rutherford, New Jersey.

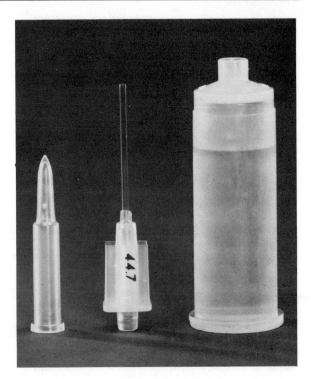

**Figure 3-11.** UNOPETTE—A collection and dilution unit for blood samples. *(Courtesy of Becton-Dickinson and Company, Rutherford, New Jersey.)*

The standard Unopette test is comprised of: (1) a disposable, self-filling diluting pipette consisting of a straight, thin wall, uniform-bore glass capillary tube fitted into a plastic holder and (2) a plastic reservoir containing a premeasured volume of reagent for diluting.

Each capillary pipette is color-coded according to capacity for quick and easy visual identification. Color-coding for all disposable self-filling Unopette capillary pipettes is as follows: 3 $\mu$l—green, 3.3 $\mu$l—gray, 10 $\mu$l—pink, 20 $\mu$l—yellow, 25 $\mu$l—blue, and 44.7 $\mu$l—black.

## Transporting Microspecimens

Glycolysis in red blood cells and white blood cells causes a decrease in blood pH which can be detected after a blood gas sample has been at room temperature for approximately 20 minutes. Therefore, blood gas microsamples should be immersed in ice water from time of collection until delivered to the clinical laboratory. Plastic containers that are small enough to hold these specimens with ice should be carried on the specimen collection tray. Ice is usually available on the patient ward. Other items to be carried on a microcollection tray include:

1. alcohol or Betadine pads,
2. marking pens for labels,

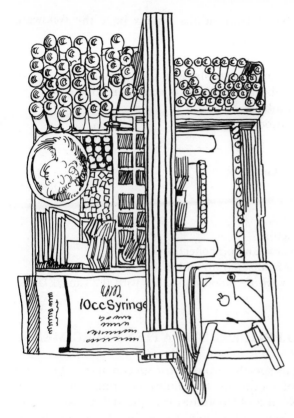

**Figure 3-12.** Specimen collection tray. *(Courtesy of College of American Pathologists (CAP), Skokie, Illinois.)*

3. Microtainer blood serum separator tubes, 600 μl,
4. Microtainer capillary whole blood cell collectors with 0.23 mg EDTA, 200 μl,
5. lancets for skin puncture,
6. sterile gauze pads,
7. unheparinized plastic microcentrifuge tubes,
8. heparinized plastic microcentrifuge tubes, 250, 400 and 500 μl,
9. heparinized Natelson tubes, 75 μl,
10. Unopettes for collection and dilution procedures.

## SPECIMEN COLLECTION TRAYS

The phlebotomist needs a specimen tray (Fig. 3-12) to take on blood collecting rounds. The tray should include all necessary collection equipment and usually differs from one hospital or clinic to another depending upon the patient population. For example, if the phlebotomist works in a children's hospital, he or she needs microcollection trays as described earlier.

Phlebotomists that collect blood from adults usually have the following equipment on their trays:

1. marking pens,
2. vacuum tubes (sterile and nonsterile) with the anticoagulants designated in the clinical laboratory blood collection manual,
3. holders for vacuum tubes,
4. needles for vacuum tubes and syringes,
5. syringes,
6. tourniquet,
7. alcohol, iodine, or Betadine pads,
8. sterile gauze pads,
9. bandages,
10. dispensers for needles,
11. lancets for skin puncture,
12. Unopettes for fingerstick blood collection,
13. Microtainer blood serum separator tubes, 600 $\mu$l,
14. Microtainer capillary whole blood collectors with 0.23 mg EDTA, 200 $\mu$l.

## TRANSPORTING AND PROCESSING PATIENT SPECIMENS

Every hospital or clinic has its specific protocol for specimen transport and process. For special types of specimens, the clinical laboratory has special handling steps. For example, if a phlebotomist is requested to transport to the laboratory an arterial specimen for blood gases, then he or she should be aware that the specimen must be transported in an airtight heparinized syringe and packed in ice. The airtight container and the ice decreases the loss of gases from the specimen. Speed is essential to avoid loss of gases from the blood.

Because glycolytic action from the blood cells interferes in chemical analysis of various chemical analysis (i.e., glucose, phosphorus, enzymes), the blood samples should be transported to the clinical laboratory as soon as possible so that the serum or plasma can be separated from the blood cells. The serum or plasma that is separated from the cells must be handled according to the laboratory procedure, therefore they may remain at room temperature, be refrigerated, stored in a dark place, or be frozen depending upon the prescribed laboratory method.

Some chemical constituents in blood such as bilirubin are light sensitive and decrease in value if exposed to light. Thus, blood collected for chemical analysis should be kept away from bright light.

Blood specimens for microbiology need to be transported to the laboratory as quickly as possible so that the blood can be transferred to culture media.

Processing specimens may occur in one location of the clinical laboratory or in each section (hematology, clinical chemistry, clinical immunology, blood bank, coagulation) dependent upon the organization of the laboratory. The phlebotomist must learn the processing requirements of the clinical laboratory so that specimens are transported and processed as quickly as possible. Efficient processing of the specimens leads to better clinical laboratory results and thus better patient care. In many laboratories, the specimen collection area has a medical technologist or medical laboratory technician who centrifuges the specimens and makes the appropriate aliquots for each section. These aliquots are then distributed to the clinical laboratory sections for testing. Some specimens must be prepared for shipping to referral laboratories. This preparation sometimes involves special packaging requirements such as freezing the specimen to maintain stability and packaging it in a styrofoam mailing container. The phlebotomist should learn the clinical laboratory task in which he or she can assist the technologist/technician in enhancing the efficiency of specimen processing.

## STUDY QUESTIONS

The following questions may have one or more answers.

1. Which of the following anticoagulants prevents coagulation of blood by removing calcium through the formation of insoluble calcium salts?

    **a.** EDTA
    **b.** ammonium oxalate
    **c.** sodium citrate
    **d.** sodium heparin

2. Which of the following anticoagulants is found in a green stoppered blood collecting vacuum tube?

    **a.** EDTA
    **b.** ammonium oxalate
    **c.** sodium citrate
    **d.** sodium heparin

3. Which of the following proteins is found in plasma, but not in serum?

    **a.** albumin
    **b.** fibrinogen
    **c.** fibrin
    **d.** globulins

4. Which of the following body fluids is extracted from joint cavities?

    **a.** pleural fluid
    **b.** peritoneal fluid
    **c.** synovial fluid
    **d.** pericardial fluid

5. When blood is collected from a patient with a syringe, the needle should

be removed from the syringe before transferring the blood to a tube in order to prevent:

**a.** hemoconcentration          **c.** glycolysis

**b.** hemolysis                  **d.** hemostasis

**6.** For capillary collection from newborns, a lancet with which of the following lengths should be used to avoid penetrating bone?

**a.** 2.50 mm                    **c.** 3.00 mm

**b.** 2.75 mm                    **d.** 3.25 mm

**7.** Which of the following blood chemical constituents is light sensitive?

**a.** glucose                    **c.** phosphorus

**b.** bilirubin                  **d.** blood gases

**8.** When blood is collected from a patient, the serum should be separated from the blood cells as quickly as possible to avoid:

**a.** hemoconcentration          **c.** glycolysis

**b.** hemolysis                  **d.** hemostasis

## REFERENCES

1. Garza D: Urine collection and preservation, in Ross DL, Neely AE (eds): Textbook of Urinalysis and Body Fluids. New York, Appleton-Century-Crofts, 1983, p 61.
2. Free AH, Free HM: Urinalysis in Clinical Laboratory Practice. Cleveland, CRC Press, 1975, pp 21–25.
3. Tietz N (ed): Fundamentals of Clinical Chemistry. Philadelphia, W.B. Saunders, 1976, pp 52–53.
4. Sunderman FW: Drug interference in clinical biochemistry. Crit Rev Clin Lab Sci 1:427, 1970.
5. Meites S: Calcium (fluorometric). Stand Meth Clin Chem 6:207, 1970.
6. Romano AT: Automated glucose methods: Evaluation of glucose oxidase–peroxidase procedure. Clin Chem 19:1152, 1973.
7. Neely WE: Simple automated determination of serum or plasma glucose by a hexokinase/G6PD method. Clin Chem 18:509, 1972.
8. Garb S: Clinical Guide to Undesirable Drug Interactions and Interferences. New York, Springer, 1971.
9. El-Dorry HF, Medina H, Bacila M: Interference of phenothiazine compounds in colorimetric determination of inorganic phosphate. Anal Biochem 47:329, 1972.
10. Hansten PD: Drug Interactions. Philadelphia, Lea and Febiger, 1981.

11. Lubran M: The effects of drugs on laboratory values. Med Clin N Amer 53: 211, 1969.
12. Sigh HP, Herbert MA, Gault MA: Effect of some drugs on clinical laboratory values as determined by the Technicon SMA-460. Clin Chem 18:137, 1972.
13. Sapira JD, Klaniecki T, Ratkin G: Non-phenochromocytoma. JAMA 212:2243, 1970.
14. Sherlock S: Progress report: Hepatic reaction to drugs. Gut 20:634–648, 1979.
15. Mettler FA: Manifestations of drug toxicity. Curr Prob In Diag Radiol 13(4): 1–55, 1979.
16. College of American Pathologists: Standards for Accreditation of Medical Laboratories. Skokie, Illinois, 1974.
17. Scranton PE: Practical Techniques in Venipuncture. Baltimore, Williams and Wilkins, 1977, p 66.
18. Standard Procedures for the Collection of Diagnostic Blood Specimens by Skin Puncture: PSH-4, NCCLS, 771E. Lancaster Ave., Villanova, PA 19085, 1977.
19. Meites S (ed): Pediatric Clinical Chemistry. Washington, D.C., The American Association for Clinical Chemistry, 1981, pp 17–19.
20. Young DS, Pestaner LC, Gibberman V: Effects of drugs on clinical laboratory tests. Clin Chem 21, 1D-4320, 1975 (special issue).

# CHAPTER 4

# Collection Procedures and Physiologic Complications

Diana Garza

## BLOOD COLLECTION

In preparing for blood collection, each phlebotomist generally establishes a routine that is comfortable for him or her. However, several essential steps go into every successful collection procedure. This chapter discusses the following steps in the same sequential manner one would progress through the blood collection process.

1. Assessing the patient's physical disposition.
2. Identifying the patient and samples.
3. Finding a puncture site.
4. Preparing the equipment, the patient, and the puncture site.
5. Performing skin or venipuncture.
6. Collecting the sample in the appropriate container.
7. Recognizing complications associated with phlebotomy.
8. Assessing criteria for sample recollection and/or rejection.

## PHYSICAL DISPOSITION

### Basal State
It is recommended that blood specimens for determining the concentration of body constituents such as (glucose, cholesterol, triglycerides, electrolytes, and proteins) be collected when the patient is in a basal state,

i.e., in the early morning approximately 12 hours after the last ingestion of food. Laboratory test results on basal state specimens are more reliable because normal values are most often determined from specimens collected during this time. Several factors such as diet, exercise, emotional stress, diurnal variations, posture, tourniquet application, and chemical constituents (drugs), cause changes in the basal state. For information on chemical substances that interfere with laboratory results, see Chapter 3.

## Diet

To ensure that the patient is in the basal state, an overnight fast is necessary. Before collecting a specimen, it is recommended that the phlebotomist ask the patient if he or she has eaten. Blood composition is significantly altered after meals and consequently is not suitable for many clinical chemistry tests. If the patient has eaten, and the physician still needs the test, it is informative if the words "NON-FASTING" are written on the requisition form.[1]

Inadequate patient instructions are often the cause of mistakes in specimen collection. The phlebotomist may be asked to explain diet restrictions to a patient. In such cases, it is necessary to explain the fasting restrictions clearly and in detail. Written instructions can be given, if available. Gaining the patient's understanding and cooperation is important and is determined by the attitude and degree of confidence displayed by the phlebotomist. Casual instructions are apt to be taken lightly by the patient or even forgotten. A phlebotomist who is organized, attentive, skilled, and who emphasizes important points of the procedure is more likely to get patient cooperation, an accurate test result, and make the patient more comfortable. If a procedure involves some discomfort or inconvenience, the patient should be informed. For example, if timed blood glucose levels are to be drawn, the patient needs to fast for 12 to 14 hours. The phlebotomist can inform the patient that several specimens will be collected at timed intervals and that he or she may drink water but coffee and tea should be avoided because they cause a transitory fluctuation in the blood sugar level. Similarly, some patients assume that the term "fasting" refers to abstaining from food *and* water. Abstaining from water can result in dehydration which can also alter test results.

Normally, serum is clear, light yellow, or straw colored. Turbid serum appears cloudy or "milky" and can be due to bacterial contamination or high lipid levels in the blood. It is caused primarily by ingestion of fatty substances such as meat, butter, cream, and cheese. If a patient has recently eaten these substances, he or she may have a temporarily elevated lipid level and the serum will appear "lipemic" or cloudy. Lipemic serum does not represent a basal state and a note on the requisition form about the appearance may be useful to the physician. Some chemical abnormalities may be indicated by lipemic serum.

## Exercise

Muscular activity, as a result of moderate or excessive exercise, has a marked effect on laboratory results such as lactic acid, creatinine, fatty acids, some amino acids, proteins, and some enzymes. Most of these values, except for certain enzymes, return to baseline levels shortly after stopping the exercise. However, enzymes such as creatine phosphokinase (CPK), aspartate amino transferase (AST), and lactate dehydrogenase (LDH) can remain elevated even after 24 hours following 1 hour of moderate to strenuous exercise.[2]

## Stress

Patients are often frightened, nervous, and overly anxious. These emotional stresses can cause a transient elevation in WBCs, transient decrease in serum iron, and abnormal adrenal hormone values.[1,2] Newborn infants who have been crying violently will display WBC counts 140 percent above resting baseline counts. Even mild crying has been shown to increase WBC counts 113 percent. These elevated counts return to baseline values within 1 hour. It is recommended that blood samples for WBC counts be taken after approximately 1 hour has elapsed.[3] Anxiety which results in hyperventilation also causes acid–base imbalances, increased lactate, and increased fatty acids.[2]

## Diurnal Rhythms and Posture

Diurnal rhythms are body fluid fluctuations during the day. Certain hormone levels are decreased in the afternoon while eosinophil counts and serum iron levels are elevated.

Posture changes are known to vary laboratory results of some constituents. This is an important consideration when comparing inpatient and outpatient results. Changing from supine (lying) position to a sitting or standing position causes body water to shift from intravascular to interstitial compartments (in tissues). Certain larger molecules are not filterable into the tissue, therefore, they become more concentrated in the blood. Enzymes, proteins, lipids, iron, and calcium are significantly increased with changes in position.[2]

## Other Factors Affecting the Patient

Many other factors can affect laboratory results. Age, gender, and pregnancy have an influence on laboratory testing. Normal reference values are often noted according to age.

Geographical location, i.e., altitude, temperature, and humidity, also affect normal baseline values. Therefore, it is important that each clinical laboratory establish normal reference values for their own population of patients and their location.

## IDENTIFICATION

### Patient Identification

Hospitalized patients should wear an identification bracelet indicating their name and designated hospital number (often called a "unit number"). Hospital unit numbers help distinguish patients with the same first and/or last names. Upon entering the room, the phlebotomist should ask the patient what is his or her name. If one asks "Are you Ms. Doe?" an ill patient on medication may mistakenly answer yes, so it is best to ask "What is your name?" and let the patient reply. Prior to any specimen collection, the patient *must* be correctly identified by his/her identification bracelet. Information on the bracelet may also include the patient's room number, bed assignment, and physician (Fig. 4-1). If the patient does not have an identification bracelet, the nurse responsible for the patient must be asked to make the identification. Documentation of the situation and the nurse's name should be made on the requisition form. It is recommended that specimens not be collected until a positive identification can be made. Blood drawn from a misidentified patient is an action for which one may be counseled, and/or dismissed.

### Specimen Identification and Labeling

Specimens should be labeled at the patient's bedside and consistently include the following information (see Fig. 4-1):

1. Patient's full name
2. Hospital unit number
3. Date of collection
4. Time of collection
5. Phlebotomist's initials
6. Patient's room number and/or bed assignment is optional information.

The phlebotomist may confirm all the information before leaving the patient's hospital room or before drawing another clinic outpatient. It is recommended that tubes *NOT* be prelabeled. Identification mistakes can easily be made if prelabeled tubes are not used, then inadvertently picked up for use on another patient. The date and time are necessary because requisition forms may indicate the date and time a laboratory test was *ordered,* rather than the date and time it was *collected.* In timed specimens, i.e., glucose tolerance, the actual collection time is critical to the test. The phlebotomist's initials are necessary to help clarify questions about the specimen if any arise during laboratory processing or testing.

There is no foolproof method for labeling specimens. The phlebotomist may write directly on the container. Many commercial collection tubes have an affixed blank label for this purpose. However, capillary tubes,

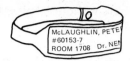

**A.** Sample identification bracelet. Printed information should include: patient's name, hospital number, room number, patient's physician.

| | | HAPPY HOSPITAL<br>DEPARTMENT OF LABORATORY MEDICINE | | DATE REQUESTED _3/17/84_ TIME REQUESTED _7:15_ |
|---|---|---|---|---|

**TEST REQUEST SLIP**

| TEST | RESULT | PERFORMED BY |
|---|---|---|
| | | |
| | | |
| | | |
| | | |
| | | |
| | | |
| | | |
| | | |

DATE REQUESTED _3/17/84_   TIME REQUESTED _7:15_

DATE COLLECTED _3/17/84_   TIME COLLECTED _7:15_

NAME ___Peter McLaughlin___

ADDRESS ___4129 University Blvd.___

___Houston, Texas___

PATIENT ROOM NO. _1708_   BED NO. _1_

AGE _34_   SEX _M_   HOSPITAL I.D. NO. _60153-7_

PHYSICIAN ___Dr. Nemitz___

TODAY ☐     ROUTINE ☐

EMERGENCY ☐     SIGNED _DMW_

**B.** Sample requisition form.

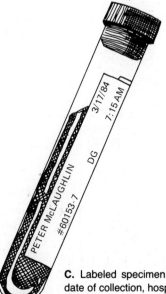

**C.** Labeled specimen. Printed information should include: patient's name, date of collection, hospital unit number, time of collection, phlebotomist's initials.

**Figure 4-1.** Identification bracelet, requisition, labeling. *(Adapted from Valaske MJ (ed): So You're Going to Collect a Blood Specimen, ed 2. Skokie, Illinois, College of American Pathologists, 1982, with permission.)*

microcollection tubes and vials, or other containers without labels must be identified either by labeling them directly with a permanent felt-tip pen, by wrapping an adhesive label around them, or by placing them into a larger labeled test tube for transport. In some cases, computerized adhesive labels with printed information are available with and detachable from the requisition form.

Laboratory requisition forms must contain the following information[4] (see Fig. 4-1):

1. Patient's full name
2. Hospital unit number
3. Date of collection
4. Time of collection
5. Collector's initials
6. Room number
7. Physician's name

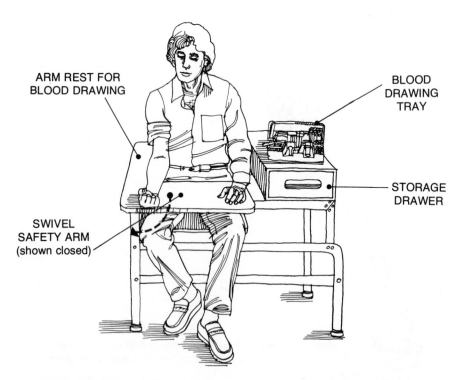

**Figure 4-2.** Equipment and patient positioning. *(Courtesy of College of American Pathologists, Skokie, Illinois.)*

## PERFORMING THE PHLEBOTOMY

It is important to choose the least hazardous site for blood collection by skin puncture or venipuncture. Several techniques can facilitate the selection of a suitable site.

### Positioning of the Patient and Venipuncture Sites

Proper positioning is important to both the phlebotomist and the patient for a successful venipuncture or skin puncture. Efforts to make sure that the patient is comfortable are worthwhile. Patients should not stand or sit on high stools because of the possibility of fainting. A reclining position is preferred, however, sitting in a sturdy, comfortable chair with arm supports is also acceptable (Fig. 4-2). The phlebotomist can position him or herself in front of the chair to protect the patient from falling forward if he or she faints. A slight rotation of the arm or hand may help expose a vein and keep it from rolling as the needle is inserted. A pillow may be used for arm support of a bedridden patient. Equipment should be placed in an accessible spot where it is not likely to be disturbed by the patient.

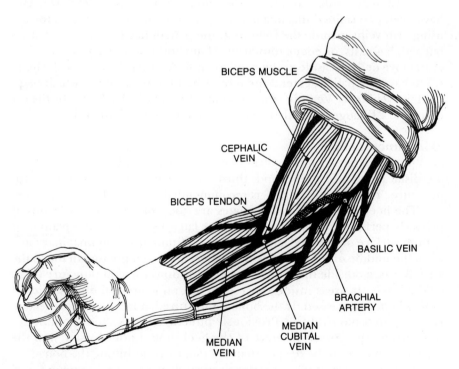

**Figure 4-3.** Veins of the anterior surface of the arm. *(Courtesy of American College of Pathologists, Skokie, Illinois.)*

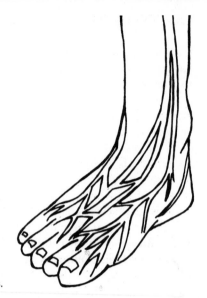

**Figure 4-4.** Foot and ankle veins.

Wrist, hand, ankle, and foot veins should be used only after arm veins have been determined unsuitable (Figs. 4-3, 4-4, and 4-5). Reasons for not using arm veins include the following: the patient has IVs in both arms, is burned, has casts, or edematous arms. Hand and foot veins have a tendency to move or "roll" aside as the needle is inserted therefore it may be helpful to have the patient extend the foot or hand into a position which helps hold the vein taut. Venipuncture in small veins may be facilitated by the use of a 19 to 21 gauge butterfly needle, as mentioned in Chapter 3.

### Skin Puncture Sites
Skin puncture most often involves one of the fingers. The fleshy surface of the distal portion of the second, third, or fourth fingers can be used for puncture. The "middle finger" is recommended.

The heels of infants and neonates are good sites for skin puncture if properly performed. The most medial or lateral sections of the plantar or bottom surface of the heel should be used. If one draws an imaginary line from the middle of the great toe to the heel and from the fourth toe to the heel, the area outside these lines is least hazardous for skin puncture (Figs. 4-6 and 4-7). If areas inside this region are punctured, the possibility of hitting bone is increased. If the bone is punctured, it may become infected, resulting in osteomyelitis.[3] Previously punctured sites should not be repunctured; the posterior curve of the heel should not be used; and the puncture should not be deeper than 2.4 mm to avoid hitting the bone.[5]

The thumb, great toe, or earlobe are rarely used as sites for skin puncture. Swollen or edematous areas should not be used for venipuncture or skin puncture because body fluids can contaminate the specimen.

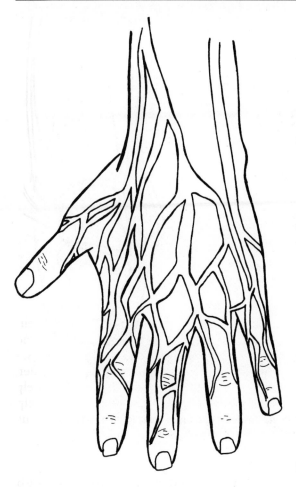

**Figure 4-5.** Wrist and hand veins.

## Warming the Site

Warming the site helps facilitate phlebotomy by increasing arterial blood flow to the area. Although several methods for warming are available, surgical towels or a wash cloth heated with warm water to 42 degrees will not burn the skin. When wrapped around the site for 3 to 10 minutes, the skin temperature can increase several degrees. The wrap can be encased in a plastic bag to help retain heat and keep the patient's bed dry.

## Tourniquet Application

A tourniquet or blood pressure cuff may be used to help find a site for phlebotomy. A soft rubber tourniquet about 1 inch (2.5 cm) wide and about 18 inches (45 cm) long is most comfortable. To apply it the ends should be stretched around the arm, both ends can be held in one hand while the

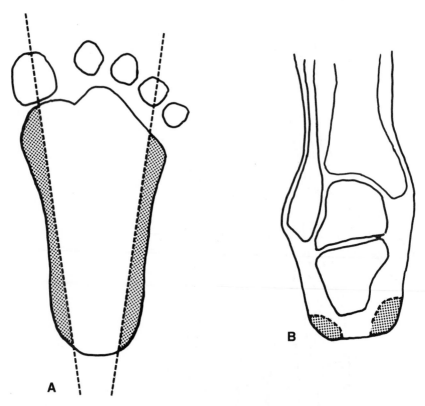

**Figure 4-6.** Heel puncture sites. **A.** The least hazardous areas for skin puncture are outside the dotted lines. **B.** Posterior view of heel and bones.

other hand grasps the area next to the skin and makes a partial loop with the tourniquet. It should be tight but not painful to the patient (Fig. 4-8). The partially looped tourniquet should allow for easy release during the venipuncture procedure. It should not be left on for more than about 60 seconds because it becomes uncomfortable and causes hemoconcentration, i.e., increased blood concentration of large molecules such as proteins, cells, and coagulation factors. Patients may be asked to clench and unclench their fist a *few* times. Excessive clenching also results in hemoconcentration. If no vein surfaces, the patient may be asked to dangle the arm for 1 to 2 minutes, then the tourniquet may be reapplied and the area palpated again.

### Decontamination of the Site
Once the site has been selected, it should be decontaminated with a sterile swab or sponge soaked in alcohol; 70 percent isopropanol is recommended (refer to Fig. 4-8).

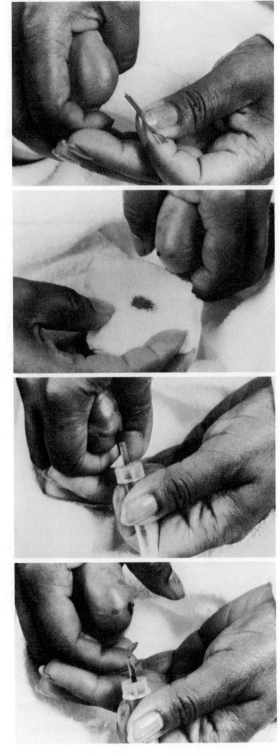

**Figure 4-7.** Performing a heel puncture. *(Courtesy of Becton-Dickinson and Company, Rutherford, New Jersey.)*

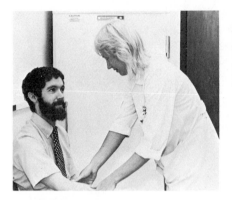

**A.** Greeting the patient.

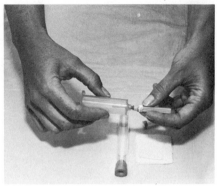

**B.** Equipment preparation.

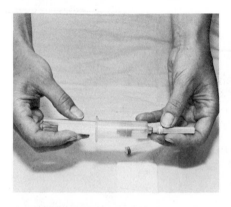

**C.** Equipment preparation.

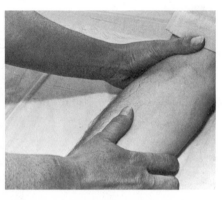

**D.** Site selection: Inspecting the site.

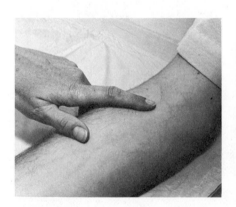

**E.** Site selection: Palpating the site.

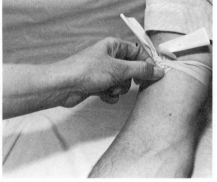

**F.** Tourniquet application.

**Figure 4-8.**

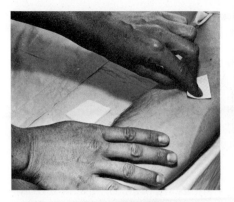

**G.** Decontamination with alcohol.

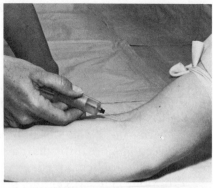

**H.** Entering the vein.

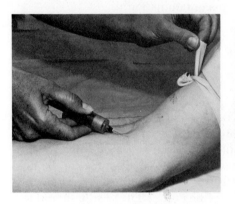

**I.** Venipuncture and removal of tourniquet.

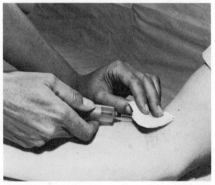

**J.** Tube and needle removal.

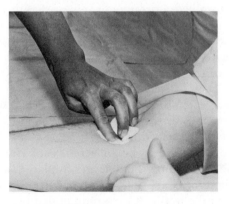

**K.** Applying pressure.

The site should be rubbed vigorously with the alcohol sponge. Some recommend rubbing in concentric circles working from the inside out. The phlebotomist should decontaminate his or her own fingers if he or she intends to palpate the site again. The decontaminated area should not be touched with any nonsterile object. Alcohol should be allowed to dry or wiped off with sterile gauze or cotton after preparing the site, otherwise it will sting at the puncture site and can interfere with test results, i.e., blood alcohol levels. When doing a finger stick, if alcohol is not wiped dry with sterile gauze, the blood will not form a round drop, therefore making microcollection more difficult. It also causes misleading cell counts because red blood cells are hemolyzed.

Providone iodine (Betadine) preparations are primarily used for drawing blood gases and blood cultures (refer to Chapter 5). For some patients, iodine causes skin irritations. Efforts should be made to remove iodine from the skin with sterile gauze after decontamination.

## METHOD OF VENIPUNCTURE AND SKIN PUNCTURE

### Venipuncture

Once the area has been cleansed, the patient's arm may be held below the site, pulling the skin tightly with the thumb. A syringe, butterfly, or Vacutainer assembly can be used for venipuncture. (Before inserting the needle, if a syringe is used, the plunger should be moved back and forth to allow for free movement and to expel all air.) The whole assembly can be held between the thumb and the 3rd or 4th finger. (The index finger may rest on the hub of the needle to guide the needle entry.) The needle should run the same direction as the vein and should be inserted at approximately a 15° angle with the skin. The needle should be inserted with the bevel site upwards and directly above a prominent vein or slightly below the palpable vein. It may be necessary to palpate with one hand after needle insertion if the vein has not been hit. Often the phlebotomist can feel a slight "pop" when the needle enters the vein. As the blood begins to flow, the patient may open his or her fist. The tourniquet can be released immediately or after the blood has been collected, but before needle withdrawal.

If a Vacutainer system is used, the test tube should be pushed *carefully* into the holder, thereby puncturing the test tube cap with the inside needle and allowing blood to enter the evacuated tube. (Refer to Figs. 3-3 and 4-8.) If multiple sample tubes are to be collected, each tube should be *gently* removed from the Vacutainer holder and replaced with another tube. Experienced phlebotomists are able to mix a full tube in one hand while waiting for another tube to fill. It is recommended that tubes for coagulation studies be filled last to avoid contamination by tissue coagulation factors released during needle insertion. (Refer to Chapter 5 for further discussion.)

If a syringe is used, the plunger can be drawn back slowly until the required amount of blood is drawn. Care must be taken not to accidentally withdraw the needle while pulling back on the plunger, or not to pull hard enough to cause hemolysis or collapse of the vein.

After tourniquet release and collection of the appropriate amount of blood, the entire needle assembly should be withdrawn quickly. A sterile, dry gauze or cotton ball should be applied with pressure to the puncture site for several minutes or until bleeding has ceased. If the patient has a free hand, he or she may apply the pressure. The arm may be kept straight, bent at the elbow, or elevated above the heart. (Refer to Fig. 4-8.)

If a syringe has been used, the blood should be quickly transferred to the appropriate test tubes to avoid clotting in the syringe barrel. This can be accomplished by using evacuated test tubes. The needle may be inserted into the tube allowing blood to be suctioned into the tube. Blood forced into the tube may cause damage to or hemolysis of cells. It is often recommended that the needle and the tube cap be removed before transferring the blood from the syringe to the test tube to avoid hemolysis. All anticoagulated specimens should be *gently* mixed by inverting 10 to 12 times.

Figures 4-9, 4-10, 4-11, and 4-12 describe specific laboratory procedures used to do venipuncture, skin puncture (fingerstick), and nursery collection, respectively. All laboratories should have phlebotomy procedures which have been approved by both the clinical laboratory supervisor and the laboratory director.

### Skin Puncture

Microcollection by skin puncture involves many of the same steps as venipuncture. The site should be cleansed as was indicated. If performing a heel stick, the infant's heel should be held with a firm grip, forefinger at the arch of the foot and thumb below and away from the puncture site, i.e., at the ankle as indicated in Figure 4-7. If doing a finger stick, the finger should be held firmly with the thumb away from the puncture site (refer to Fig. 4-11). The puncture should be done in one sharp continuous movement almost perpendicular to the site and across the fingerprint. If the puncture is made along the lines of the fingerprint, blood has a tendency to run down the finger. Average depth of a skin puncture should be 2 to 3 mm. In heel sticks on infants, the depth should not exceed 2.4 mm.[5,6] Special lancets, which control the depth of the puncture, are available commercially. Pressure from the phlebotomist's thumb may be eased and reapplied as the drops of blood appear. Massaging or milking the area should not be done because it causes hemolysis and contamination of tissue and intracellular fluids into the blood specimen.[5]

## Procedure

1. Knock on the patient's door and enter the room.
2. Introduce yourself as being from the laboratory and needing to collect a blood sample, which the doctor has ordered.
3. After presumptively identifying the patient by bed labels or by asking for him or her by name, ask the patient his or her full name (if the patient is conscious and competent to respond).
4. In all cases, check the patient's identification armband to verify that the request slip and the armband are identical. If the patient is not wearing an armband or if the armband and the request slip are not identical, report the situation to the nurse, who must provide a correct armband before the blood is drawn. If it is impossible, for physical reasons, to attach an armband to the patient or if it is a request for stat work on a new patient who does not have an armband, have the nurse write on the request slip, "ID by _____ (nurse's name)."
5. Prepare tubes and needle-holder assembly and place beside the patient before the tourniquet is applied.
6. Select site on arm for venipuncture, after placing the tourniquet several inches above the elbow. *Blood may not be drawn from a site above an intravenous infusion, but must be obtained from a site on the patient's other arm if necessary.*
7. Cleanse the site with an alcohol prep and allow it to air-dry before you enter the vein. Drying may be assisted by fanning the area with your hand. Do not blow on the site.
8. Puncture the vein and obtain proper tubes for the tests ordered. The tourniquet should be removed at the first sign of blood flow to prevent blood stasis at the puncture site.
9. Remove the needle from the vein, and immediately apply pressure to the site with clean 2″ × 2″ gauze. The patient may apply pressure with the other hand, or if that is impossible, the blood collector should apply pressure for 2 to 3 minutes. The patient should not be instructed to bend his or her arm up, as this reopens the puncture site and may cause damage to the vein and surrounding tissue.
10. Tubes containing anticoagulants must be mixed promptly and may be inverted with one hand while the other applies pressure if the patient is unable to assist.
11. When the bleeding stops, label the tubes properly with the patient's first and last name, unit number, date, and time of collection and initials before leaving the bedside. Collector's initials, date, and time must be written on top of the request slip using a ballpoint pen or permanent felt tip pen. If the patient has been applying pressure to the puncture site, remove the gauze and check the site for bleeding. Never leave the room until bleeding has stopped. If necessary, call the nurse for assistance.
12. Wash your hands immediately before leaving the patient's room especially if you have had skin contact with the patient's blood or other biologic fluid.
13. Thank the patient, and leave the room, after checking the area to be sure that all used equipment has been removed. Return to the nursing station to initial and time the log book opposite the patient's name.

## Quality Control

1. Strict adherence to procedures is essential, because without a properly obtained blood specimen, test results will not be meaningful to the physician.
2. Tubes containing anticoagulants must be inverted promptly after blood is drawn. When several tubes are drawn, tubes containing anticoagulants should be filled last.
3. When coagulation studies are ordered, the blue top vacutainer tubes containing sodium citrate should be drawn after filling at least one other tube to prevent entry of tissue thromboplastin into the tube. This substance will affect results of the coagulation tests. *(continued)*

4. Avoid prolonged application of the tourniquet. If a vein is not located in a minute or two, release the tourniquet for 1 to 2 minutes, then retie and look again, or look on the other arm. Prolonged obstruction of the vein will lead to false results for some tests.
5. Never attempt more than two venipunctures on a patient if you are unable to obtain the blood. Give the patient and yourself a fresh start with someone else.
6. Never dispose of needles in a wastebasket in the patient's room. Dispose of them in a special area in the laboratory. All needles should be clipped in a Destructoclip before replacing needle cap.
7. Never prelabel blood tubes. If blood is not obtained on that patient, the tubes may be mistakenly used on a different patient.
8. Always provide proper information on the request slips and blood tubes. If there are any questions about the specimen, it is important to be able to contact the collector. It may also be necessary to interpret test results, so the time the specimen was drawn is vital information.

---

Clinical Laboratory Supervisor                          Laboratory Director

**Figure 4-10.** Performance of a fingerstick. *(Adapted from University of Texas Department of Pathology and Laboratory Medicine, Hermann Hospital, Houston, Texas, with permission.)*

**Procedure**
1. Choose a finger that is not cold, cyanotic, or swollen. If possible, the stick should be at the tip of the fourth or ring finger of the nondominant hand.
2. Gently massage the finger five or six times from base to tip to aid blood flow.
3. With an alcohol swab, cleanse the ball of the finger.
4. Allow to air-dry.
5. Remove the lancet from its protective paper without touching the tip.
6. Hold the patient's finger firmly with one hand and make a swift, deep puncture with the lancet halfway between the center of the ball of the finger and its side.
7. The cut should be made across the fingerprints to produce a large, round drop of blood.
8. Wipe the first drop of blood away with a clean gauze.
9. Gently massage the finger from base to tip to obtain the proper amount of blood for the tests requested.
10. Each type of micro sample has different collection tube and blood volume requirements.

**Notes**
If the patient's hands are cold, wrap one of them in a warm to hot towel 10–15 minutes before the puncture is performed.

**Quality Control**
A free-flowing puncture is essential to obtain accurate test results. Do not use excessive squeezing to obtain blood.

---

Clinical Laboratory Supervisor                          Laboratory Director

88

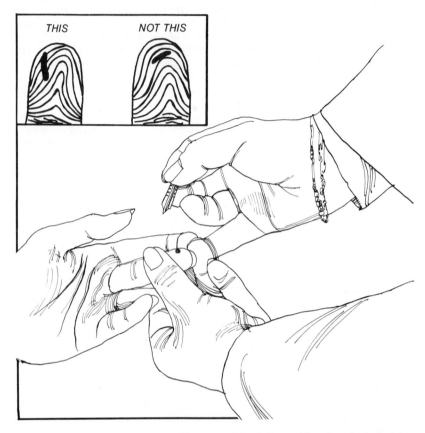

**Figure 4-11.** The finger puncture. *(Courtesy of the College of American Pathologists, Skokie, Illinois.)*

**Figure 4-12.** Nursery procedure. *(Adapted from the University of Texas Department of Pathology and Laboratory Medicine, Hermann Hospital, Houston, Texas, with permission.[3])*

**Principle**

To obtain blood specimens from infants with the least amount of trauma while maintaining good isolation techniques.

**Procedure**

1. The entrance to the nurseries (intensive care, intermediate care, and low risk) is located on _____.
2. Place blood collection tray on the table near the scrub sinks outside the nurseries.
3. Remove rings, watches, and lab coat.  *(continued)*

4. Wash hands with regular soap. The water is controlled using foot pedals.
5. Put on a gown with ties in the back. If your clothes have long sleeves, wear a yellow paper gown. With short sleeves, wear a short-sleeved cotton gown.
6. Scrub hands thoroughly using the following technique:
   a. Turn on water and wet hands.
   b. Using prepackaged brushes impregnated with soap, scrub hand, nails, and lower arms for 3 minutes.
   c. Rinse hands thoroughly.
   d. Dry hands with paper towel.
   e. Turn off faucet with paper towels.
7. Pick up tray with two clean paper towels and enter nursery area.
8. Find the small metal cart and place tray on a clean diaper on the cart.
9. Discard paper towels.
10. Identify the baby by making sure the request slip is identical to the baby's armband.
11. After ensuring the skin is warm, perform a heel puncture to obtain the proper blood specimen for the tests requested.
12. Hold a clean cotton gauze over the puncture site until bleeding stops. Do not put Band-Aids on the baby's feet.
13. Remove all collection equipment from the crib to avoid harming the baby.
14. Before collecting blood from the next baby, wash hands at the sink inside the nursery proper.
15. Initial the log book for all work completed.
16. Remove gown and discard in proper receptacle.
17. Wash hands.
18. When moving from one nursery area to the other, the blood collector must repeat the complete scrub technique and put on a clean gown.

**Notes**
1. The baby's heel may be punctured a maximum of two times. Do not stick a baby more than twice to obtain a specimen at any given time. If a particular baby must always be punctured the maximum number of times, notify the supervisor of specimen control and the baby's primary nurse.
2. Do not puncture a foot if there are bruises, abrasions, or sloughing skin present. Call this to the attention of the baby's nurse.
3. To help obtain a free-flowing puncture wound from a baby who doesn't bleed freely, have a nurse wrap the baby's heel in a warm towel 10 to 15 minutes before the puncture is made. This is also necessary for collection of all capillary blood gases.
4. Use only gentle massage when obtaining blood. Excessive massaging dilutes the blood with tissue fluids and may also cause hemolysis. It is sufficient to massage with your thumb and forefinger.
5. Never repuncture old puncture wounds.
6. *Never* remove a baby from its isolette or change its position in any way without the approval of a nurse.
7. Collect specimens from babies in isolation for an infectious disease last to avoid any risk of spreading the disease to other infants. Take only the equipment you need into an isolation room. Everything but the blood specimen must be discarded in the room. Follow approved isolation technique.
8. Any employee with a respiratory infection or skin lesions on hands must not be allowed to have patient contact.

---

Clinical Laboratory Supervisor

Laboratory Director

The first drop of blood should be removed with a sterile dry pad. Capillary tubes, i.e., Unopette, and blood smears can then be made from subsequent drops of blood.

Figures 4-13 and 4-14 indicate methods for making blood smears and blood dilutions with capillary pipets. Figure 4-15 demonstrates use of the Microtainer system. The phlebotomist should remember that alcohol prevents round drops from forming. Care must be taken when filling capillary tubes not to get air bubbles into the tube. This leads to erroneous results for many laboratory tests.

All disposable equipment should be discarded in appropriate containers. Paper and plastic wrappers can be thrown in a waste basket. Needles and lancets should *not* be thrown in a waste basket, but in a sturdy disposable container to be autoclaved.

Before leaving the patient's side, the phlebotomist should check the site to make sure that the bleeding has stopped. All tubes should be appropriately labeled and confirmed. All supplies and equipment brought in should be removed.

An adhesive bandage may be applied. However, they are not recommended for infants or young children because of possible irritation and the potential of swallowing or aspirating a bandage.[3]


## COMPLICATIONS AND SPECIAL CONSIDERATIONS IN BLOOD COLLECTION

### Fainting (Syncope)
Many patients become dizzy and faint at the thought or sight of blood. It is important to be aware of the patient's condition throughout the collection procedure. This can be done by verbal communication. If a seated patient feels faint, the needle should be removed and the head lowered between the legs and the patient should breathe deeply. Talking to patients can often reassure them and divert their attention from the collection procedure. Patients in bed rarely feel faint. In both cases, however, the phlebotomist should stay with the patient till he or she recovers. A wet towel gently applied to the forehead or a glass of juice or water may help the patient feel better.

### Failure to Draw Blood
Several factors may cause one to "miss the vein" such as not inserting the needle deep enough, inserting the needle all the way through the vein, holding the needle bevel against the vein wall, or losing the vacuum in the tube (Fig. 4-16). The phlebotomist's index finger can help locate the vein while the needle is inserted. It may be necesssary to move or withdraw the needle somewhat, and redirect it. On occasion, a test tube will have no vacuum because of a manufacturer's error or tube leakage after a puncture. It

# THE BLOOD SMEAR

Blood smears can be made either from venous blood or from capillary (finger) blood. In each case, the smears should be made from fresh blood and not anticoagulated blood.

**CAPILLARY METHOD:**

1. Make a finger puncture in the usual way and wipe away the first drop of blood.

2. Touch the slide to the second drop of blood and transfer a small drop of it to the slide about one-half inch from one end.

3. Hold the slide containing the drop of blood in your left hand. With your right hand, place the end of a second slide, balanced on the finger tips at an angle no greater than 30 degrees, in front of the drop of blood.

4. Pull the spreader slide back into the drop of blood. When the blood has spread along two-thirds of the width of the slide, push the spreader slide forward with a steady even motion. The weight of the slide is the only downward pressure applied.

5. Allow the smear to air dry. DO NOT BLOW ON IT!!

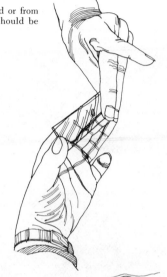

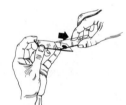 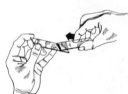 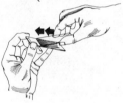

**A GOOD SMEAR SHOULD MEET THE FOLLOWING CONDITIONS:**

a. The entire smear should cover no more than one-half of the area of the slide.

b. No portion of the smear should extend to the edges of the slide.

c. There should be no ridges, lines, or holes in the smear.

**THE ERRORS TO AVOID ARE:**

a. Too large a drop of blood.

b. Too long a delay in transferring the drop of fresh blood to the slide and making the smear.

c. Using a spreader slide with a chipped or unpolished end.

d. Delay in making the smear, allowing the blood drop to dry on the finger.

**USING VENOUS BLOOD:**

Immediately after removing the needle from the vein, touch the tip of the needle gently to a slide to produce a drop one to two mm in diameter. Then proceed as outlined in the above procedure.

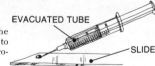

EVACUATED TUBE

SLIDE

**Figure 4-13.** This illustrates preparation of a thin film of blood on a glass slide. *(Courtesy of the College of American Pathologists, Skokie, Illinois.)*

**Figure 4-14.** Blood dilutions using capillary pipets. *(Courtesy of Becton-Dickinson and Company, Rutherford, New Jersey.)*

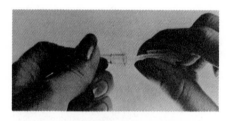

**1.** Puncture diaphragm: Using the protective shield on the capillary pipette, puncture the diaphragm of the reservoir as follows:
a. Place reservoir on a flat surface. Grasping reservoir in one hand, take pipette assembly in other hand. Push tip of pipette shield firmly through diaphragm in neck of reservoir, then remove.

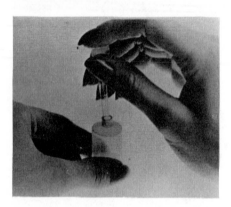

b. Remove shield from pipette assembly with a twist.

**2.** Add sample
Fill capillary with sample and transfer to reservoir as follows:
a. Holding pipette *almost* horizontally, touch tip of pipette to sample. Pipette will fill by capillary action. Filling is complete and will stop automatically when sample reaches end of capillary bore in neck of pipette.
b. Wipe excess sample from outside of capillary pipette, making certain that no sample is removed from capillary bore.

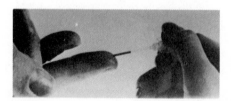

*(continued)*

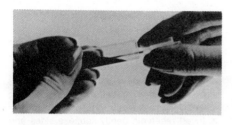

c. Squeeze reservoir slightly to force out some air. Do not expel any liquid. Maintain pressure on reservoir.

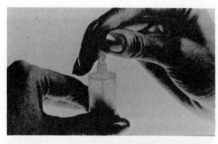

d. Cover opening of overflow chamber with index finger and seat pipette *securely* in reservoir neck.

e. Release pressure on reservoir. Then remove finger from pipette opening. Negative pressure will draw blood into diluent.

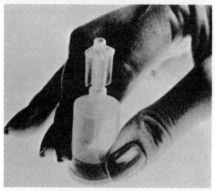

f. Squeeze reservoir *gently* two or three times to rinse capillary bore, forcing diluent into, *but not out of,* overflow chamber, releasing pressure each time to return mixture to reservoir. CAUTION: If reservoir is sequeezed too hard, some of the specimen may be expelled through the top of the overflow chamber.

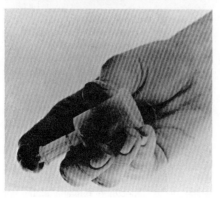

g. Place index finger over upper opening and gently invert several times to thoroughly mix sample with diluent. *(continued)*

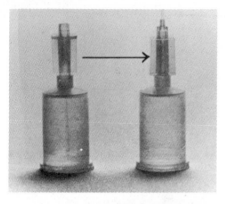

**3.** Count cells (option 1)
Mix diluted blood thoroughly by inverting reservoir (see 2g) to resuspend cells immediately prior to actual count.
a. Convert to dropper assembly by withdrawing pipette from reservoir and reseating securely in reverse position.
b. Invert reservoir, gently squeeze sides and discard first three or four drops.
c. Carefully charge hemacytometer with diluted blood by gently squeezing sides of reservoir to expel contents until chamber is properly filled.

OR

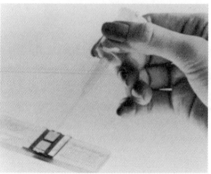

**3.** Transfer contents (option 2)
Transfer thoroughly mixed contents of each reservoir to appropriately labeled test tubes or corresponding cuvettes as follows:
a. Convert reservoir to dropper assembly by withdrawing pipette and reseating securely in reverse position as shown above.

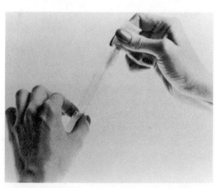

b. Place capillary tip into appropriately labeled test tube or cuvette which will accommodate 5.0 ml of reagent and squeeze reservoir to expel entire contents.

OR

**3.** Store diluted specimen (option 3)

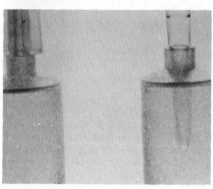

Cover overflow chamber with capillary shield or remove capillary and insert tip of shield firmly into reservoir opening. (Note time for which diluted specimen remains stable for each test.)

behooves the phlebotomist to carry an extra set of tubes in his or her pocket in case this happens during venipuncture. Also, needles for evacuated tube systems have been known to unscrew from the barrel during venipuncture. If this happens, the tourniquet should be released immediately and the needle removed.

## Hematomas

When the area around the puncture site starts to swell, this usually indicates that blood is leaking into the tissues causing a hematoma. This can happen when the needle has gone completely through the vein, the bevel opening is partially in the vein, or when not enough pressure is applied to the site after puncture (refer to Fig. 4-15). If a hematoma begins to form, the tourniquet and needle should be removed immediately and pressure applied to the area.

## Petechiae

These are small red spots appearing on a patient's skin which indicate that minute amounts of blood have escaped into skin epithelium. This may be a result of coagulation problems, i.e., platelet defects, and should caution the phlebotomist that the patient's puncture site may bleed excessively.

## Edema

Some patients develop an abnormal accumulation of fluid in the intercellular spaces of the body. This swelling can be localized or diffused over a larger area of the body. The phlebotomist should avoid collecting blood from these sites because veins are difficult to palpate or stick, and the specimen may be contaminated with fluid.

## Obesity

Obese patients generally have veins that are difficult to visualize and palpate. If the vein is missed, the phlebotomist must be careful not to probe excessively with the needle because it causes rupture of RBCs, increased concentration of intracellular contents, and releases some tissue clotting factors.

## IV Therapy

Patients on IV therapy for extended periods of time often have veins which are palpable and visible but are damaged or occluded (blocked). Every time a catheter is used, vein damage occurs. Circulatory blood is rerouted to collateral veins and can result in hemoconcentration.

In cases where a patient has an IV line, that arm should not be used for venipuncture because the specimen will be diluted with IV fluid. The other arm, or another site, should be considered. It is sometimes possible for the nurse or physician to disconnect the IV line and draw blood from the needle that is already inserted. The first few ccs of the specimen should be dis-

**Figure 4-15.** How to collect capillary blood using the Microtainer system. *(Courtesy of Becton-Dickinson and Company, Rutherford, New Jersey.)*

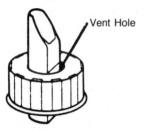

Vent Hole

**A.** Flotop collector.

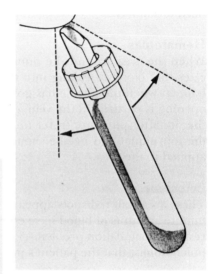

**B.** Collect blood.

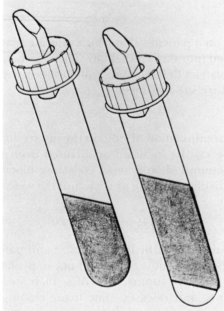

**C.** Fill serum tubes.

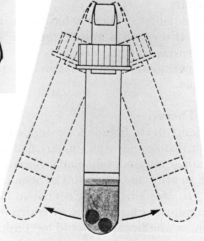

**D.** Fill EDTA tubes.

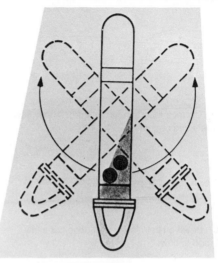

**F.** Cap and invert EDTA tubes.

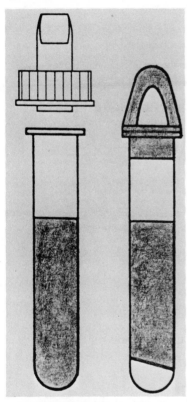

**E.** Cap serum tubes.

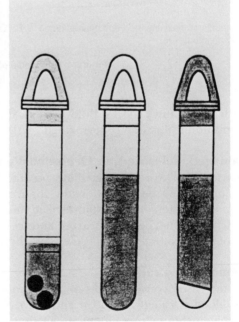

**G.** Transport tubes.

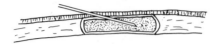

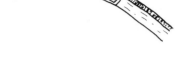

**A.** Correct insertion technique; blood flows freely into needle.

**B.** Bevel on vein upper wall does not allow blood to flow.

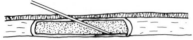

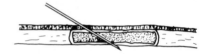

**C.** Bevel on vein lower wall does not allow blood to flow.

**D.** Needle inserted too far.

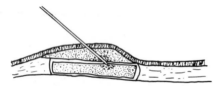

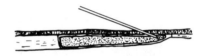

**E.** Needle partially inserted and causes blood leakage into tissue.

**F.** Collapsed.

**Figure 4-16.** Needle positioning.

carded to remove the IV fluid. A note should be made on the laboratory requisition if this step is performed.

### Damaged, Sclerosed, or Occluded Veins
Veins, which are obstructed or occluded, do not allow blood to flow through. Sclerosed or hardened veins are a result of inflammation and disease of the interstitial substances. Patients' veins that have been repeatedly punctured often becomes scarred and feel very hard when palpated. Blood is not easily collected from these sites, therefore they should be avoided.

### Hemoconcentration
An increased concentration of larger molecules and formed elements in the blood is called hemoconcentration. Several factors can cause this to happen including tourniquet application, massaging, squeezing or probing a site, long-term IV therapy, and sclerosed or occluded veins.

## Hemolysis

When RBCs are lysed, hemoglobin is released and serum (normally straw color) becomes tinged with pink or red. If a specimen is grossly hemolyzed, the serum appears very dark red. Hemolysis can be caused by improper phlebotomy techniques such as using a needle that is too small, pulling a syringe plunger back too fast, expelling the blood vigorously into a tube, and shaking or mixing tubes vigorously. These problems can easily be prevented by appropriate handling. Hemolysis may also be the result of physiologic abnormalities. The phlebotomist should make a note on the requisition form when he or she notices that a specimen is hemolyzed.

## Collapsed Veins

If a syringe plunger is withdrawn too quickly during venipuncture, it may cause the vein to collapse. This is especially true when collecting blood from the smaller veins (refer to Fig. 4-16).

## Allergies

Some patients are allergic to iodine or other solutions used to disinfect a site. If a patient indicates that he or she is allergic to a solution, all efforts should be made to use an alternative method.

## Thrombosis

Thrombi are solid masses derived from blood constituents which reside in the blood vessels. A thrombus may partially or fully occlude a vein (or artery) making venipuncture more difficult.

## Burned or Scarred Areas

Areas that have been burned or scarred should be avoided during phlebotomy. Burned areas are very sensitive and susceptible to infection. Veins under scarred areas are difficult to palpate.

## Infections

The phlebotomist should remember at all time that many patients have transmittable diseases, i.e., hepatitis. A phlebotomist, in turn, can pass an infection to a patient. (For precautionary techniques, see Chapter 6.)

## RECOLLECTION

Each hospital or clinic should establish guidelines and policies for specimen rejection and recollection. A recollection policy should include the following information:

1. The number of times a patient can be punctured by the same phlebotomist. Generally, a phlebotomist should not puncture a patient
   more than twice before calling for a second opinion.
2. The number of times a patient can be punctured in one day. It is
   recommended that staff physicians, nurses, and medical technologists coordinate their efforts to minimize patient venipuncture.
3. The volume of blood that can be drawn daily from a patient,
   especially in pediatrics and the nursery (Table 4-1).

Because the health-care team (including doctors, medical technologists, clerks, secretaries, and nurses) are all working for the welfare of the
patient, they should strive to reduce the number of phlebotomies. Several
suggestions for doctors, nurses, ward clerks, and laboratory personnel have
been given to do this.

Doctors could write orders on the same line on the chart rather than
scattered throughout a page. Orders can be coordinated among all the staff
physicians working with the patient. Notification to the laboratory of multiple timed tests ordered would be helpful. If a patient needs a hemoglobin

**TABLE 4-1. MAXIMUM AMOUNTS OF BLOOD TO BE DRAWN ON PATIENTS UNDER 14 YEARS**

| Patient's Weight | | Maximum Amount to Be Drawn at Any One Time | Maximum Amount of Blood (Cumulative) During a Given Hospital Stay (1 Month or Under) |
|---|---|---|---|
| Pounds | kg (approx) | | |
| 6-8 | 2.7-3.6 | 2.5 ml | 23 ml |
| 8-10 | 3.6-4.5 | 3.5 ml | 30 ml |
| 10-15 | 4.5-6.8 | 5 ml | 40 ml |
| 16-20 | 7.3-9.1 | 10 ml | 60 ml |
| 21-25 | 9.5-11.4 | 10 ml | 70 ml |
| 26-30 | 11.8-13.6 | 10 ml | 80 ml |
| 31-35 | 14.1-15.9 | 10 ml | 100 ml |
| 36-40 | 16.4-18.2 | 10 ml | 130 ml |
| 41-45 | 18.6-20.5 | 20 ml | 140 ml |
| 46-50 | 20.9-22.7 | 20 ml | 160 ml |
| 51-55 | 23.2-25.0 | 20 ml | 180 ml |
| 56-60 | 25.5-27.3 | 20 ml | 200 ml |
| 61-65 | 27.7-29.5 | 25 ml | 220 ml |
| 66-70 | 30.0-31.8 | 30 ml | 240 ml |
| 71-75 | 32.3-34.1 | 30 ml | 250 ml |
| 76-80 | 34.5-36.4 | 30 ml | 270 ml |
| 81-85 | 36.8-38.6 | 30 ml | 290 ml |
| 86-90 | 39.1-40.9 | 30 ml | 310 ml |
| 91-95 | 41.4-43.2 | 30 ml | 330 ml |
| 96-100 | 43.6-45.5 | 30 ml | 350 ml |

(Adapted from Becan-McBride K: Textbook of Clinical Laboratory Supervision, New York, Appleton-Century-Crofts, 1982, with permission.)

at 2 PM and a glucose at 3 PM, it may be possible to coordinate the times and draw both specimens with one venipuncture.[7]

Nurses and ward secretaries could organize laboratory orders as much as possible to avoid sending frequent requests minutes apart. When transcribing orders, all of them should be requested at the same time. The laboratory should be notified of patient transfers. An up-to-date log of room numbers and patients' names should be available on the ward as a resource for laboratory personnel.

Laboratory personnel should organize requisition forms by patient and by floor. Any identification discrepancies should be communicated to a nurse.[7]

One hospital has suggested several slogans for their health care personnel regarding phlebotomy:[7]

A stick in time saves nine.
We care—several pokes are no joke.
For their sake, let's stick together.

## SPECIMEN REJECTION

Each department or section in the clinical laboratory should establish their own guidelines for rejection of a specimen. Generally speaking, the following factors should be considered: discrepancies between requisition forms and labeled tubes (names, dates, times), unlabeled tubes, hemolyzed specimens (except in tests where it does not interfere), specimens in the wrong collection tubes, use of outdated equipment, supplies, or reagents, and contaminated specimens.

When a problem arises, the appropriate investigational channels should be followed. The phlebotomist who drew the specimen and his or her supervisor should try to solve the problem initially. Other personnel may be involved as needed. Communication and honesty are the keys to an efficient and reliable hospital environment.

## STUDY QUESTIONS

Choose one or more of the following answers.

1.  Normal laboratory values are calculated from which type of specimen:

    **a.** basal state          **c.** random samples during the day
    **b.** early morning       **d.** evening

2.  A patient may be identified by which of the following means:

    **a.** patient's chart          **c.** patient's armband
    **b.** nurse                     **d.** ward clerk

3.  Which of the following is *"not"* a site for skin puncture:

    **a.** wrist      **c.** ankle
    **b.** vein       **d.** heel

4.  When is it beneficial to use a "butterfly needle"? For:

    **a.** heel puncture               **c.** veins in the ankle
    **b.** veins in the wrist or hand  **d.** fingerstick

5.  What effect does warming the site have on venipuncture?

    **a.** it keeps veins from rolling   **c.** it causes hemoconcentration
    **b.** it makes veins stand out      **d.** it increases localized blood flow

6.  What is the best angle for needle insertion during venipuncture?

    **a.** 15°      **c.** 45°
    **b.** 30°      **d.** 80°

7.  Why is it necessary to control the depth of lancet insertion during skin puncture? To avoid

    **a.** puncturing a vein          **c.** excessive bleeding
    **b.** bacterial contamination    **d.** osteomyelitis

8.  Which of the following factors result in failure to draw blood during venipuncture?

    **a.** losing the vacuum in the tube   **c.** needle was inserted through
    **b.** tourniquet is on too tight          the vein
                                           **d.** veins are sclerosed

9.  Hematomas during venipuncture result from which of the following:

    **a.** needle bevel is against the vein wall       **c.** needle is occluded
    **b.** needle bevel is partially inserted in the   **d.** patient has coagulation
       vein                                               problems

10. Hemoconcentration can be caused by which of the following:

    **a.** long-term IV therapy          **c.** excessive needle probing
    **b.** lengthy tourniquet application **d.** sclerosed or occluded veins

# REFERENCES

1. Damon Corporation: Handbook of Specimen Collection and Preparation, Damon Co., 1977.
2. Henry JB: Todd, Sanford, Davidsohn-Clinical Diagnosis and Management by Laboratory Methods. Philadelphia, W.B. Saunders, 1979, p 15.
3. Becton-Dickinson: Blood Specimen Collection by Skin Puncture in Infants. Becton-Dickinson Vacutainer Systems, Rutherford, NJ, 1982.
4. Becan-McBride K: Textbook of Clinical Laboratory Supervision. New York, Appleton-Century-Crofts, 1982.
5. Meites S, Levitt MJ: Skin puncture and blood collecting techniques for infants. Clin Chem 25:183−189, 1979.
6. Lilien LD, Harris VJ, Ramamurthy RS, Pildes RS: Neonatal osteomyelitis of the calcaneus: Complications of heel puncture. J Pediatrics 88:478−480, 1976.
7. Larson JM: A stick in time saves nine. MLO, April, pp 109−117, 1981.

# CHAPTER 5
# Special Tests and Collection Procedures

Karen Hlavaty

## SPECIAL TESTS

Depending on the specific needs of individual clinical settings, phlebotomists may be required to perform a variety of special tests or procedures in addition to routine skin tests and venipuncture. The following section presents basic techniques and precautions for various "special" tests. It is suggested that extensive training sessions and supervision accompany the student phlebotomist in these procedures because they can harm the patient if performed incorrectly.

### Arterial and Capillary Blood Gases

Arterial blood is the specimen of choice for testing the pH, oxygen ($O_2$), and carbon dioxide ($CO_2$) content of the blood. As discussed in a preceding chapter, skin puncture blood is less desirable as a specimen source because it contains blood from capillaries, venules, arterioles, and fluids from the surrounding tissue. In addition, common collection methods for "capillary" blood gases employ an open collection system in which the specimen is temporarily exposed to room air, theoretically allowing for a brief exchange of gases (both $O_2$ and $CO_2$) before sealing the specimen from the air.

Capillary blood gases are often collected from small children and babies for whom arterial punctures can be too dangerous. They are collected from the same areas of the body as other capillary samples such as the lateral posterior area of the heel, the great toe, or the ball of the finger. (Refer to Chapter 4 for microcollection procedures.)

When a capillary blood gas is ordered, the phlebotomist should warm the area well ahead of time to ensure that a good blood flow is obtained and that blood can be quickly collected, anticoagulated, and sealed from contact with room air. To do this procedure, a site is chosen and a cloth or diaper is saturated with warm water and wrapped around the foot or hand for 5 to 10 minutes. Care should be taken that the warming cloth is not too hot; if the warmed diaper or cloth can be held comfortably in the hand, it is not too warm for the baby. When the phlebotomist is prepared to collect the blood gas, the cloth should be removed and the area dried. The puncture site should be cleaned and entered in the usual manner for all skin punctures (as discussed in Chapter 4). A heparinized capillary (Fig. 5-1) tube with a volume of at least 100 $\mu l$ should be used to collect the specimen. A metal filing may be inserted into the tube before collecting to help mix the specimen while it is entering the tube. It is extremely important that the specimen be collected with no air bubbles which can distort the values obtained from the specimen. When the tube is full, the ends should be sealed with plastic caps or clay (according to the individual laboratory protocol) and a magnet should be used to draw the metal filing back and forth across the length of the tube to completely mix the specimen. The tube should then be submerged in an ice bath for transfer to the laboratory. The skin puncture site should be pressed with a clean gauze sponge until bleeding stops and a bandage may be left over the spot.

## Arterial Blood Gases

When an arterial blood gas is ordered, the experienced phlebotomist, nurse, or physician should palpate the areas of the forearm where the artery is typically close to the surface, namely, the brachial artery in the cubital fossa and the radial artery in the radial sulcus of the forearm. If the arms of the patient cannot be used, the femoral artery in the groin may be

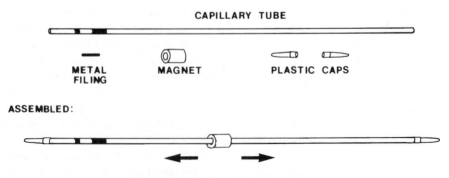

**Figure 5-1.** Capillary blood gas tubes.

used. With the forefinger or first two fingers, the phlebotomist should press at these sites in order to find the artery. The thumb should never be used for palpating because there is a pulse in the thumb that may be confused for the patient's own pulse.

Once the site is decided upon, the area should be cleaned well with povidone–iodine solution (Betadine). No tourniquet is required as the artery has its own strong blood pressure. As in venipuncture, a syringe with needle can be used to withdraw the sample. The addition of a small amount of liquid heparin to coat the syringe barrel will anticoagulate the blood. The phlebotomist should pull the skin taut and enter the pulsating artery at a high angle, usually no less than 45 degrees. Little or no suction is needed as the blood flows quickly into the syringe under its own pressure. When enough sample has been drawn (usually about one milliliter), the phlebotomist withdraws the needle, applies gauze and direct manual pressure on the site for at least 15 minutes. The syringe should be quickly capped and placed in ice *immediately* in an effort to keep the blood gases from escaping into the atmosphere. Ideally the specimen should be analyzed within ten minutes of collection, therefore, immediate transport of the specimen to the laboratory is advised. Before leaving the patient, the phlebotomist should clean the puncture site with an alcohol pad to remove the excess Betadine and a pressure bandage should be left on. If bleeding from the site persists, the phlebotomist should apply more manual pressure and ring for assistance from the patient's nurse. The phlebotomist should never leave a patient who is bleeding, particularly after an arterial puncture. The primary nurse should be notified after an arterial puncture is performed so that the area may be checked frequently for deep or superficial bleeding.

## Bleeding Time—Duke and Ivy Methods

The bleeding time is a useful tool for testing platelet plug formation in the capillaries. It is generally used in conjunction with other coagulation tests for diagnosing coagulopathies or problems in hemostasis.

The Duke method measures the time from incision to cessation of bleeding at the ear lobe site. It is difficult to standardize and does not allow for ample surface area to repeat the test when necessary. If bleeding is excessive, it is difficult to control at this site. It may also be noted that testing on the ear lobe may cause undue apprehension in the patient because he/she cannot observe the procedure. For these reasons, the Duke method is not commonly recommended and will not be discussed.

The Ivy method is the preferred method. It assesses bleeding time by utilizing the volar surface of the forearm for testing. The length and depth of incision can be standardized with a commercial template. This site allows ample surface area to conduct repeat tests. If bleeding becomes excessive, it can be controlled readily.

When a bleeding time is ordered, the phlebotomist must be sure that the patient has not taken aspirin or drugs containing salicylates within the previous two weeks, as it has been shown to interfere with platelet plug formation for up to two weeks. If the patient's platelet count is less than 100,000/cu mm, the bleeding time may be prolonged.

The phlebotomist should begin the procedure by explaining the process to the patient and asking him or her to relax his/her arm. The sphygmomanometer cuff can be applied to the upper arm and inflated to a pressure of 40 mm Hg. This pressure should be maintained throughout the procedure. The volar surface should be cleaned with alcohol and prepared as for a venipuncture. A site that is free of surface veins or visible capillaries, scars, tattoos, or hair should be selected. Using the template, two incisions can be made as close together as possible without allowing the blood flow to overlap. Starting a stopwatch, the blood drops that form at the incisions should be blotted gently at 30 second intervals. Care should be taken that the blood is not wiped away as the platelet plug may be disturbed and cause the bleeding time to be prolonged. The blood should be merely absorbed onto the filter paper by touching the tip of the drop. If bleeding becomes excessive between intervals, a sterile gauze pad can be used to wipe away blood that has traveled beyond the incisions.[3]

The stopwatch is stopped when bleeding has ceased from both incisions. The cessation of bleeding from the two sites should vary by no more than 30 seconds. If the difference in time is greater than 1 minute, a repeat should be considered. Normal values are generally considered to be 1 to 6 minutes, though ranges may vary slightly among different institutions.

After the test time is noted on the request slip, the phlebotomist should deflate the pressure cuff and apply a bandage to the incisions. If the bleeding has not stopped within 15 minutes, the stopwatch may be stopped and the time noted on the request slip as "greater than 15 minutes." The pressure cuff should be removed and manual pressure applied to the site. As in all cases, the phlebotomist should remain with the patient until bleeding stops.

## Lee-White Clotting Time

This manual test is poorly reproducible, insensitive to significant coagulation factor deficiencies, and time-consuming. The Lee-White clotting time can easily be replaced by automated methods for prothrombin (PT) and activated partial thromboplastin time (PTT). For monitoring heparin therapy, it is considered obsolete at many institutions because other routine coagulation will suffice.

## Microbiologic Cultures

Specimens for microbial culture are often transported to the laboratory by phlebotomists. Most of them have been collected using sterile equipment and procedures. These specimens are screened in the microbiology laboratory for the presence of infectious agents such as bacterial parasites, fungi, and viruses. The phlebotomist should recognize the potential hazards in handling these specimens and the need for maintaining them in sterile containers. If a phlebotomist inadvertently contaminates one of these specimens, it may lead to false positive results which can be harmful to the patient.

Phlebotomists are asked most often to collect blood cultures. Occasionally, a phlebotomist may be asked to collect other specimens for culture such as swabs of the throat or nasopharynx, and urine. Regardless of the source, the phlebotomist should check hospital policies before practicing such procedures. If a health-care facility does allow phlebotomists to collect these specimens, he or she should be thoroughly familiar with the procedures before attempting them on a patient.

## Blood Cultures

Blood cultures are often collected on patients who have fevers of unknown origin (FUO). Sometimes, during the course of a bacterial infection, bacteremia may result and become the dominant clinical feature. In the case of a patient who experiences fever spikes, it is generally recommended that blood cultures be drawn before and after the spike, when bacteria may be most likely present in the peripheral circulation. It is best to draw one set of aerobic and anaerobic cultures at the time the order is given. Thirty minutes later, a second set of anaerobic and aerobic cultures should be obtained. A request for "second site" blood cultures that are obtained concurrently on opposite arms is useful when the physician suspects bacteremia due to a local, internal infection. However, a "second site" culture is *not* a very effective tool for *routine* blood culture orders and provides relatively little information that properly spaced, timed blood cultures cannot provide.[4]

When an order is received for a blood culture, the phlebotomist should briefly explain the procedure to the patient and make an effort to alleviate any visible apprehension. As with a routine venipuncture, the phlebotomist should apply the tourniquet and locate a suitable site on the arm. The tourniquet should then be released while "prepping" the arm. The site and surrounding area should be scrubbed well with surgical green soap for 2 minutes. If the phlebotomist feels that the area needs to be repalpated before sticking, he or she should clean his or her forefinger in exactly the same manner as the patient's arm or use a sterile glove.

After scrubbing with the soap, a sterile alcohol pad is used to wipe away the soap from the site of puncture. It should be wiped moving outward in increasing concentric circles. The alcohol must be allowed to dry in order to kill surface bacteria. Then, povidone–iodine solution in a presoaked pad or a commercial applicator should be applied, starting from the puncture site and moving out and away from the center (Fig. 5-2). This solution must also be allowed to dry in order to be effective against surface bacteria. During this final drying period, the tourniquet may be reapplied and the tops of the blood culture bottles may be cleaned with sterile alcohol pads. A syringe and needle or evacuated tube assembly is prepared cautiously so as not to exercise the plunger, destroy the sterility, or eliminate the anaerobic conditions of the syringe. A second needle should be readily available. The venipuncture is performed in the usual manner. The tourniquet is released and the needle withdrawn; sterile gauze is quickly placed over the site and the patient should be asked to apply pressure to the site with the other hand.

The used needle should be destroyed, removed from the syringe, and replaced with a large, clean needle for delivery into the culture bottles (Fig. 5-3). These bottles contain a nutrient broth. Most hospitals inoculate at least two blood culture bottles from each site, one for aerobic and another for anaerobic incubation. The anaerobic culture bottle should be filled first and the aerobic culture bottle second. Changing needles prior to inoculating the bottles eliminates bacterial contamination from the pores and deep recesses of the tissue which may be picked up as the needle is removed from the site. Some blood culture bottles are shaped to fit into the barrel apparatus just as an evacuated tube would, therefore, eliminating one step (Fig. 5-4). After inoculating the bottles, the surrounding puncture site should be cleaned with alcohol to remove the iodine on the skin. A bandage may be placed over the site when the bleeding has stopped. As in all collected specimens, the bottles should be clearly marked with the appropriate information. (Refer to Chapter 4.) Figure 5-5 is an actual hospital procedure for collection of blood cultures.

## Throat and Nasopharyngeal Culture Collections

Nasopharyngeal cultures are often performed to detect carrier states of *Neisseria meningitidis, Corynebacterium diphtheriae, Streptococcus pyogenes, Haemophilus influenzae,* and *Staphylococcus aureus.* In children and infants,

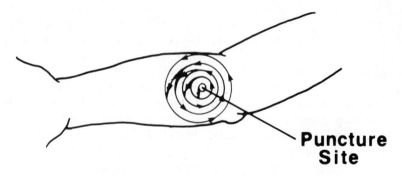

**Puncture Site**

**Figure 5-2.** Arm preparation for blood cultures.

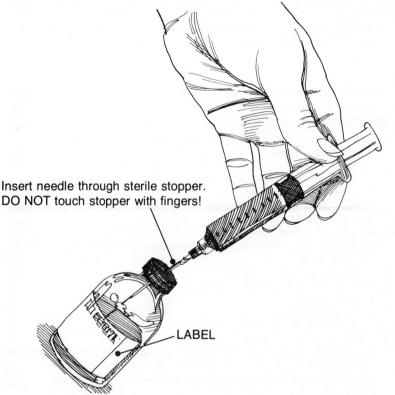

Insert needle through sterile stopper.
DO NOT touch stopper with fingers!

LABEL

**Figure 5-3.** Inoculating blood culture bottles. *(Courtesy of College of American Pathologists, Skokie, Illinois.)*

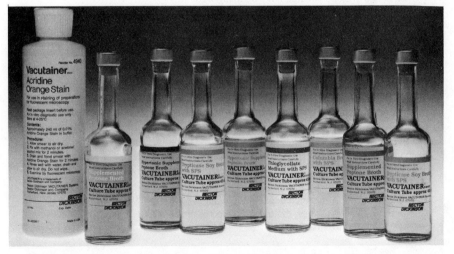

**Figure 5-4.** Vacutainer blood culture bottles. *(Courtesy of Becton-Dickinson and Company, Rutherford, New Jersey.)*

**Figure 5-5.** Collection of Blood Cultures. *(Courtesy of the University of Texas Department of Pathology and Laboratory Medicine, Hermann Hospital, with permission.)*

---

**Principle**
Prevention of contamination of the blood culture by skin organisms is the primary concern of the blood collector when obtaining blood for this test.

**Procedure**
1. Apply the tourniquet to the patient's arm and select a site for venipuncture.
2. Remove the tourniquet.
3. Preparation of the patient's arm is a three-step technique:
    a. Cleanse the site with surgical green soap (in Cepti-seals™) for 2 minutes.
    b. Remove soap using an alcohol prep.
    c. Apply iodine solution (in Cepti-seals) to the site in a particular motion, beginning at the center of the site selected for venipuncture.
4. Allow the iodine solution to air-dry. Do not touch the disinfected site of venipuncture unless the finger used for palpation is similarly disinfected or unless sterile surgical gloves are worn.
5. Reapply the tourniquet.
6. Obtain blood with a 12ml syringe and a 22 gauge or 20 gauge needle.
    a. Adult patients – 5 ml.
    b. Pediatric patients:
        (1) Children 2 to 12 years – 2 ml.
        (2) Infants under 2 years – 1 ml.
7. Inject the blood into a 50 ml bottle of BHI Broth, the top of which has been cleansed with a sterile PVP prep. Do not change needles.
8. Invert the bottle gently, and label with the usual patient identification information, and time of collection.
9. Do not insert airway into blood culture bottle.
10. After the patient's arm has stopped bleeding, remove the iodine solution by wiping with a clean alcohol prep.
11. Indicate on the request form and on the bottle which culture number you have drawn if a series of blood cultures have been ordered.
12. Blood cultures may not be ordered any less than 1 hour apart.

**Notes**
1. If the patient is known to be hypersensitive to iodine, omit the iodine cleansing step above or you may substitute methiolate.
2. Number of blood cultures is determined by clinical urgency of the situation. In most adult infections, collect three to four 5 ml samples over a period of 24 hours at intervals of at least 1 hour. Use the same protocol in patients with suspected SBE. In patients already on therapy, collect four to six samples within 4 hours at intervals spaced no closer than ½ hour. For severe clinical infections, when requested by the attending physician, collect two 5 ml samples, taken by separate venipuncture (preferably, one from each arm), immediately before medication is administered. In infants, two samples taken at intervals of at least 1 hour are usually sufficient to diagnose sepsis.

**Quality Control**
1. Do not touch the venipuncture site after it has been prepared.
2. The requisition must show the date and time collected and the initials of the collector.

from whom significant sputum cultures are difficult to obtain, naso-pharyngeal cultures may be used to diagnose whooping cough, croup, and pneumonia. Throat cultures are most commonly obtained to determine the presence of streptococcal infections.

Because coughing may force organisms from the lower respiratory tract into the nasopharynx, it may be best to perform a throat culture on a child or infant and stimulate coughing in order to obtain a more significant nasopharyngeal culture.

When a throat culture is ordered, the patient should be instructed to open the mouth wide, as if to yawn. A light source should be directed into the mouth and throat so that areas of inflammation, ulceration, exudation, or capsule formation can be readily seen. A tongue blade or spoon is used to depress the tongue and prevent contamination with organisms from the oral cavity. A sterile cotton swab should be used to brush both tonsillar areas, the posterior pharynx, and all other areas of possible infection.

The swab can then be placed in a special transport media or used to inoculate directly onto agar in a petri dish by rolling it across a small area of the media. It can then be transported to the laboratory where it may be spread out or "streaked" for distribution of the microorganisms. A Gram-stained smear is often useful to provide preliminary indications of infection and should be made with the swab by rolling it across a slide before placing it in transport media or inoculating plate agar. The slide, swab, and any inoculating media should be brought to the laboratory and processed as soon as possible after collection. The culture should be placed under opti-mal growth conditions for suspected pathogens. This is accomplished by incubating the culture. Timely processing of the specimen helps prevent overgrowth of normal flora which can inhibit or mask any pathogenic orga-nisms present.

Nasopharyngeal specimens should be obtained with a Dacron- or cotton-tipped flexible wire that can be easily sterilized prior to use. Com-mercially packaged sterilized swabs are also available. The swab is passed gently through the nose and into the nasopharynx where it is rotated, care-fully removed and then placed into transport media or inoculated onto media for isolation. Again, stress should be placed on the importance of timely processing of all specimens for very best results.

## Skin Tests
On occasion, a phlebotomist may be asked to perform a skin test. Again, the phlebotomist should check the policies of the hospital prior to perform-ing the procedure. Skin tests are simple and relatively inexpensive. They determine if a patient has ever had contact with a particular antigen and has produced antibodies to that antigen. A wide range of disease states stimulate antibody responses in individuals. Tests range from detection of ragweed and milk allergies in hypersensitive individuals, to tuberculosis

and fungal infections in persons who have had contact with these organisms.

The skin test is administered by pulling in 0.1 ml of diluted antigen into a tuberculin syringe. All air bubbles should be expelled by holding the syringe straight up and tapping the sides of the barrel. The volar surface of the forearm should be cleaned with alcohol and prepared in the same manner as for a venipuncture. (See Chapter 4 on venipuncture collection.) The area should be devoid of scars, skin eruptions, or excessive hair. Holding the syringe at a small angle (approximately 20 degrees), the needle should be slipped just under the skin. The plunger should be pulled back to ensure that a blood vessel has not been entered. The fluid may be slowly expelled into the site. The needle should be promptly removed and only *slight* pressure is applied with gauze over the site. Care should be taken that the fluid does not leak out onto the gauze or run out of the injection site. It is best that the patient remain with the arm extended until the site has had time to close and retain the fluid. A bandage should not be used over the site as it may absorb some of the fluid and may distort the results of the skin tests by causing skin irritation from the adhesive. The patient should report any reaction whatsoever to the physician. Also, a return visit for proper interpretation of the skin reaction should be scheduled with the physician.

## Glucose Tolerance Test

In patients who have symptoms suggesting problems in carbohydrate metabolism, such as diabetes mellitus, the glucose tolerance test can be an effective diagnostic tool. The test is performed by first obtaining fasting blood and urine specimens, giving the fasting patient a standard load of glucose, and obtaining subsequent blood and urine samples at intervals usually over a five-hour period. Each specimen is then analyzed for glucose content. In general, glucose levels should return to normal within two hours after ingesting the glucose. In diabetic patients, it is necessary to carry out the test for four to five hours to observe how the patient metabolizes the glucose.

When a glucose tolerance is to be performed, the patient should be given complete instructions about the procedure so his or her cooperation can be assured. For best results, the patient should eat normal, balanced meals for at least three days prior to the test. Eight to twelve hours prior to the beginning of the test, the patient should fast completely. Water intake is strongly encouraged as frequent urine specimens are required throughout the procedure. Other beverages, including unsweetened tea or coffee, are not allowed. Cigarette smoking and gum chewing (including sugarless gum) should be discouraged until the completion of the test as they may stimulate digestion and interfere with the interpretation of the results. If a patient is chewing gum prior to or during the test, note this on the requisition slip.[5]

During the test, the patient drinks a standard dose of glucose, usually 100 g in adults or approximately 1 g/kg of body weight in children and small adults. Commercial preparations are available as flavored drinks to make the glucose more palatable. The patient must start and finish the drink within 5 minutes. Water intake is encouraged throughout the procedure. If the patient should vomit at any point in the procedure, the physician should be notified immediately to decide whether the test should be continued or stopped.[5]

When the patient has finished drinking the solution, the time is noted and 30-minute, 60-minute, 120-minute, and 180-minute blood and urine specimens are obtained. In addition to the time, the tubes should be labeled "30 minutes," "1st hour," and so on (Fig. 5-6). If blood is obtained initially by venipuncture, all succeeding specimens must also be venous blood. Similarly, if capillary blood is used, all specimens should be collected by microtechnique because values and methods of analysis may vary between the two types of samples. If serum samples are used instead of plasma samples with a preservative, the tubes should be centrifuged immediately after collection, then the serum should be separated from the blood cells and placed in the refrigertaor to inhibit glucose utilization by white blood cells.

### Postprandial Glucose Test

The two-hour postprandial glucose test can be used to screen patients for diabetes because glucose levels in serum specimens drawn two hours after a

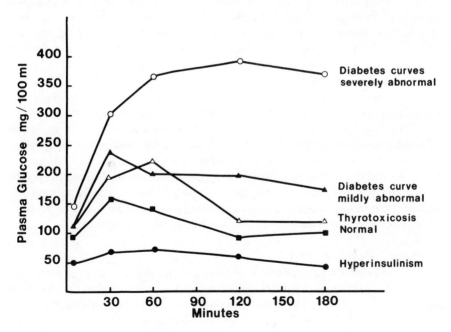

**Figure 5-6.** Glucose tolerance test.

meal are rarely elevated in normal patients. In contrast, diabetic patients will usually have increased values two hours after a meal.

For this test, the patient should be placed on a high carbohydrate diet 2 to 3 days before the test. The day of the test, the patient should eat a breakfast of orange juice, cereal with sugar, toast and milk to provide an approximate equivalent of 100 g of glucose. A blood specimen is taken 2 hours after the patient has finished eating breakfast. The glucose level on this specimen is then determined. The physician can decide if further carbohydrate metabolism tests are needed (such as a glucose tolerance test).

### Epinephrine and Glucagon Tolerance Tests

Epinephrine increases blood sugar by accelerating glycogenolysis (breakdown of glycogen). This tolerance test is used to determine availability and quantity of liver glycogen by stimulating an increase in blood sugar by epinephrine injection.

A fasting blood sugar is obtained. The physician or other qualified professional should inject 10 minims of a 1:1000 solution of epinephrine hydrochloride intravenously. Thirty minutes after the injection, another blood sample should be taken for glucose level determination. The blood sugar should rise at least 30 mg/dl at the 30 minute sample. The blood sugar level should return to the fasting level in about 2 hours. If the patient's blood sugar level does not respond or rises only slightly, several disease states may be responsible. If glycogen storage is depleted, the epinephrine has little effect and the blood sugar may rise only slightly. Such conditions exist in hepatocellular damage, such as cirrhosis and fatty liver. If glycogen stores are not readily available, though they may be present, the epinephrine has little effect on blood sugar. Von Gierke's disease is known to interfere with the availability of glycogen for conversion to sugar.

Because several disease states and possibilities exist for a low response to an epinephrine injection, this test is not considered a diagnostic tool, but used in combination with other carbohydrate metabolism studies.

The glucagon tolerance test is conducted in a similar manner as the epinephrine tolerance test. In fact, often the two stimulants may be given in combination to test liver glycogen stores. The amount of the stimulants given should be determined by the ordering physician and administered by a qualified professional or physician. The phlebotomist may be involved in drawing the blood samples for glucose determinations and may be responsible for labeling and delivering the specimens to the laboratory.

### Lactose Tolerance Test

Some otherwise healthy adults experience difficulty in digesting lactose, a milk sugar. They appear to lack a mucosal lactase enzyme that breaks down the lactose into the simple sugars, glucose and galactose. Instead, gastrointestinal discomfort may result, followed by diarrhea. These patients usually show no further symptoms if milk is removed from their diet.

To determine if a patient suffers from lactose intolerance, a physician may order a lactose tolerance test. A 3-hour glucose tolerance test should be performed one day in advance to determine the patient's normal glucose curve. A lactose tolerance test should be performed the next day in the same manner as the glucose tolerance, substituting the same amount of lactose for the glucose given the previous day. Fasting, 1-hour, 2-hour, and 3-hour blood samples are drawn and tested for glucose. The curve should be similar to that obtained in the glucose tolerance if the patient has mucosal lactase and digests the sugar properly. If the patient is intolerant to lactose, his or her blood sugar will increase by no more than 20 mg/dl from the fasting sample.

The phlebotomist should be sure that a bathroom is conveniently located to the patient testing area because patients who are lactose intolerant may experience severe discomfort during the testing.

False positive results have been known to occur in 25 to 33 percent of the patients tested who had normal lactase activity in small intestine biopsy specimens. This has been attributed to slow gastric emptying and not the absence of the lactase enzyme.

### D-xylose Tolerance Test

The D-xylose absorption test is commonly used for the diagnosis of malabsorption states. D-xylose is a pentose found in certain fruits, such as plums, but does not normally occur in the blood or urine. Therefore, a patient should be fasting before the test and instructed not to eat fruits high in D-xylose for up to three days before the test. A measured load of D-xylose is given to the patient (25 g is recommended) and then his or her urine and blood are collected to determine concentrations of D-xylose.

A 2-hour blood sample is taken and a pooled sample of urine is taken over the 5-hour period after dose administration. Both samples are analyzed for D-xylose and reported in mg/dl. Because xylose is not normally present in significant amounts in the blood, it is an excellent indicator of small intestine absorption as it passes unchanged through the liver and is excreted by the kidneys. Low values are seen in intestinal malabsorption, but are normal in pancreatic malabsorption. Low values are often obtained in cases where bacteria have overgrown in the small intestine and affected absorption in the jejunum.

### Cardio-green Dye Test

Bromsulfphalein (BSP) is a dye that has been used to test liver function. Due to the possibility of an anaphylactic response, indocyanine green (cardio-green) has been more recently the dye of choice. A patient is given a measured load of dye intravenously and a blood sample is obtained 45 minutes later and tested for the dye. Only about 5 percent of the dye should remain in normal patients.

The phlebotomist may be asked to assist in the procedure, but the physician or some other qualified person should deliver the dose intravenously. It is not recommended that a phlebotomist be responsible for the delivery of any dye, medication, or stimulant without a physician or nurse supervising. The physician should indicate the time the blood is to be collected and the phlebotomist should be responsible for seeing that the appropriate specimen is drawn and delivered to the laboratory.

## Gastric Analysis and Hollander Tests
Gastric analysis and Hollander tests determine gastric function in terms of stomach acid production. The gastric analysis measures gastric acid secretion in response to stimulation from histamine or pentagastrin, whereas the Hollander test uses insulin to stimulate gastric secretions. Both tests involve passing a tube through the patient's nose and into the stomach. Both tests require intravenous administration of either histamine or insulin. Therefore, although the phlebotomist may be asked to assist and to draw specimens as required, the responsibility for properly intubating the patient (using fluoroscopic examination) and administering the stimulant intravenously should rest with the physician or nurse. The phlebotomist can be present to assist in patient care and to draw any required blood specimens, but should under no circumstances be expected to carry out the procedure. There is high risk to the patient if the tube is improperly placed and could puncture a lung if it enters the bronchial system instead of the esophagus. The phlebotomist can and should be responsible for proper labeling of gastric and blood samples when he or she is present and assisting during the procedure.

## Sweat Chloride by Iontophoresis
The sweat chloride test is used in the diagnosis of cystic fibrosis. Patients with cystic fibrosis produce chloride in their sweat at 2 to 5 times the level produced by healthy individuals. Cystic fibrosis is a disorder of the exocrine glands, generally thought to be enzymatic in nature, which exhibits changes in mucous-producing glands in the body. Primarily affected are the lungs, upper respiratory tract, liver, and pancreas.

For the laboratory evaluation, pilocarpine-HCl hydrochloric acid (HCl) is iontophoresed into the skin of the patient to stimulate sweat production. The sweat is absorbed onto preweighed gauze pads and then the weight of the sweat is obtained. The pad is then diluted with deionized water and the chloride is generally read by titration with a chloridometer.

When a phlebotomist receives an order to perform a sweat chloride test on a patient, he or she should properly prepare for the procedure under the supervision of a medical technologist. Four cups and lids should be preweighed with two 2-inch square gauze pads in each cup. Only two cups are normally used, but the other two can be used as backups, if needed.

Choosing a site with the largest surface area (in children and infants, the leg is best suited), the phlebotomist should wipe the surface of the skin with a gauze pad soaked in deionized water. The area is wiped dry. Another 2-inch square, 8-ply gauze pad is soaked in 0.07 M sodium bicarbonate and placed on the cleaned area. The negative electrode is placed on the gauze and taped securely to the skin. The electrode should not be in direct contact with the skin at any time when the current is on.

Another gauze square is soaked in 0.33 percent pilocarpine-HCl and placed on the skin next to the sodium bicarbonate square, but not touching it. The positive electrode should be placed on that gauze and taped securely in place. Again, care should be taken that the electrode does not make direct contact with the skin at any time throughout the procedure. The area between and around the secured gauze squares should be wiped dry before the current is on. The current is turned on and very slowly raised to one milliamp. It is important that the current be increased slowly because a sudden increase may cause a shock to the patient.

After 10 minutes, the current is decreased to zero. The switch is turned off and the electrodes and gauze squares are removed. Reagent grade water is used to wipe off the pilocarpine-HCl area which is then wiped dry.

A 2 × 2-inch square of thin waxed film, such as Parafilm*, should be cut out and handled with clean forceps. Using the forceps, the film can be placed against the cleaned area and taped securely on the skin on adjacent sides. Using forceps, two gauze pads from a preweighed cup are removed and placed between the parafilm and the skin. The remaining side can be taped securely. Tape may also be applied across the top of the parafilm to prevent it from tearing. A timer should be started for one hour. During that period, the procedure should be repeated on the other arm or leg.

After one hour, the tape should be carefully removed and the gauze sponges removed with forceps and returned to the original cup. The lid must be tightly on the cup and then weighed again. After weighing, 200 $\mu l$ of deionized water should be added to the cup. The lid should be replaced and wrapped securely with parafilm. The sponges should equilibrate for 2 to 3 hours or overnight. The phlebotomist should bring the cups and the weights measured during the procedure to the laboratory where a medical technologist will measure the chloride on the chloridometer and calculate the results.[1]

## Donor Room Collections

Properly trained phlebotomists may be employed in a regional blood center or hospital blood donor center to screen and collect blood from donors. This section summarizes the procedure outlined by the American Associa-

---

*Parafilm, American Can Company, Dixie/Marathon, Greenwich, Connecticut.

tion of Blood Banks.[2] Only an experienced, properly trained phlebotomist should be considered for this function. A physical, emotional, or traumatic experience may keep a donor from volunteering in the future.

***Donor Interview and Selection.*** Not everyone who wishes to donate his or her blood is eligible. It is up to the interviewer to determine the eligibility of the donor. Carefully determining donor eligibility helps prevent the spread of disease to blood product recipients and prevents untoward effects for the potential donor.

The following information should be kept on file on every donor for at least five years and initially obtained on every prospective donor, regardless of ultimate acceptability.

1. Date of donation
2. Name: last, first and middle
3. Address
4. Telephone
5. Sex
6. Age and/or date of birth (Donors should be between the ages of 17 and 66). Minors may be accepted if written consent has been obtained in accordance with applicable law in the state.
7. Written consent form signed by the donor authorizing the blood bank to take and use his or her blood.
8. A record of reason for deferrals, if any.
9. Social security numbers or driver's license numbers may also be used for additional identification.
10. The race of a donor is not mandatory, but this information can be useful in screening patients for a specific phenotype (chromosomal makeup).

To help minimize the incidence of dizziness, fainting, or other reactions to blood loss, donors are encouraged to eat within 4 to 6 hours of donating blood. A light snack just before phlebotomy may help avoid these reactions, but a donor should not be required to eat if he or she does not wish to do so.

Blood bank records must be able to trace all components of a donor unit (RBCs, WBCs, platelets, etc.) to its disposition. If the donation is a "replacement for credit" for a particular patient, then the donor must supply the patient's name.

A brief physical examination is required to determine if the donor is in general good condition on the day he or she is to donate blood. The physical examination entails a few simple procedures easily mastered by the blood bank phlebotomist.

1. *Weight.* Donors must weigh at least 110 lb (50 kg); if their weight is less, the volume of blood donated must be carefully monitored and

care taken that not too much blood is taken; also the anticoagulant in the bag must be modified for the lesser donation. Most blood banks will not routinely accept donors who weigh less than 110 lb.

2. *Temperature.* Oral temperature must not exceed 37.5°C (99.6°F).
3. *Pulse.* It should be a regular, strong pulse between 50 to 100 beats/minute. The pulse should be taken for at least 30 seconds.
4. *Blood pressure.* The systolic blood pressure should measure 90 to 180 mm Hg and the diastolic blood pressure should be between 50 to 100 mm Hg. People outside of these limits should be deferred as donors and referred to their physicians for evaluation of a possible health problem.
5. *Skin lesions.* Both arms should be examined for signs of drug abuse such as needle marks or sclerotic veins. The presence of mild skin disorders such as psoriasis, acne, or poison ivy rash does not necessarily prohibit an individual from donating unless there are lesions in the antecubital area or the rash is particularly extensive. Donors with purulent skin lesions, wounds, or severe skin infections should be deferred. The skin at the site of the venipuncture must be free of lesions.
6. *General appearance.* If the donor looks ill, excessively nervous, or under the influence of alcohol or drugs, he or she should be deferred.
7. *Hematocrit or hemoglobin.* The hematocrit must be no less than 38 percent for female donors and no less than 41 percent for male donors. The hemoglobin value must be no less that 12.5 g/dl for female donors and no less than 13.5 g/dl for male donors. A fingerstick is commonly used to determine these values. The phlebotomist may either collect a hematocrit tube for centrifuging and reading or use the copper sulfate method in which the hemoglobin is qualitatively determined. (For further details on the copper sulfate method, please refer to the AABB Technical Manual.[2])

An extensive medical history must be taken on all potential donors regardless of the number of previous donations on record. Most blood bank donor rooms have a simple card listing all the questions to be asked and "yes" or "no" columns to check the donor's responses. Refer to the protocol of the donor room at the institution's blood bank or the AABB Technical Manual which sets guidelines for donor screening and acceptance.

***Collection of Donor's Blood.*** The phlebotomist in a donor room must operate under the supervision of a qualified, licensed physician. Blood should be collected using aseptic technique, a sterile, closed system, and a single venipuncture. If a second venipuncture is needed, an entirely new, sterile donor set is necessary; the first is discarded according to the contaminated material disposal protocol of the institution. A donor should never be left alone either during or immediately after collection of blood. The phlebotomist should be well-versed in donor reactions, equipment safety precautions, first aid techniques, and location of first aid if it should be needed in the course of donation.

The phlebotomist should prepare the antecubital portion of the donor's arm in the same manner as for collection of a blood culture specimen. (Refer to the section Special Tests, collection of blood cultures in this chapter.) The blood collecting bag should be placed conveniently and the tubing should be extended to make sure there are no kinks in the tube that would prevent a free flow. When the arm is properly prepped, the tourniquet should be replaced and the donor given instructions to open and close the hand during the course of phlebotomy. A 15-gauge "regular" or 17-gauge "thin-walled" needle is most often used. The 17-gauge thin-walled needle is preferable because it has the internal diameter of a 15-gauge needle and the outside diameter of a 17-gauge, i.e., it has the large bore size of a 15, but the smaller total size of the 17. The sterile needle is uncapped and with a quick, sure motion, the needle is slipped under the skin and into the vein. As the draw begins, the needle and tubing should be taped in place and a dry, sterile gauze sponge laid on top. The phlebotomist should encourage the donor to continue to slowly open and close the hand and to report any discomfort or dizziness if it should occur.

The phlebotomist should make sure that the blood in the bag mixes with the anticoagulant during the collection, either manually or by placing it on a mechanical agitator. If the collection process takes more than 8 minutes to complete, it is possible that platelet concentrates or antihemophilic factor preparations may not be possible. However, as long as the flow is constant and the bag contents continue to be mixed well, no time constraints are necessary.

Once the proper amount of blood has been collected (405 to 495 ml), the phlebotomy should be stopped, the tubing clamped off with a hemostat or some other temporary clamp, the tourniquet or blood pressure cuff released, the needle removed, and pressure placed over the site for several minutes. It is advisable that the donor be instructed to raise his or her arm over the head while holding the gauze with pressure over the puncture site. This method minimizes bleeding into the site and surrounding tissues as well as helps restore the integrity of the vascular tissue. The donor should not be allowed to bend the arm until bleeding stops as this may cause the tissue to be further traumatized by bleeding into the area below the skin as well as encouraging the vascular tissue to overlap and form scar tissue on the site during the healing process. A pressure bandage may be placed over the site once bleeding has stopped. The blood in the bag and tubing should be mixed well, properly labeled, and stored in accordance with blood bank standards.

The donor should be encouraged to remain seated or prostrate for 10 to 15 minutes or longer if the donor complains of dizziness or other discomfort. If the donor appears to be well, he or she should be encouraged to drink more fluids than usual to replace the volume loss and to refrain from strenuous exercise or work until after a full meal. Refreshments should be offered to the donor as a courtesy as well as in an effort to restore some of the lost body fluids. Any adverse reactions experienced by the donor should be recorded on the donor record. If the donor leaves before staff members recommend, it should also be noted on the record.

### Therapeutic Phlebotomy

Therapeutic phlebotomy is used in the treatment of some myeloproliferative diseases, such as polycythemia, or other conditions in which the removal of blood benefits the patient. Records in the Blood Bank should be kept indicating the patient's diagnosis, the physician's request for the phlebotomy, and the amount of blood to be taken. It is up to the medical director of the blood bank to decide if the patient is to be bled in the donor room or in a private section of the blood bank. Some patients are visibly ill and weak and may have some psychologic effects on healthy donors present. When a patient is obviously ill, his or her physician or the medical director of the blood bank, should be present during the phlebotomy. Generally, the patient should be bled more slowly than a healthy donor and the resting period should be extended.

The blood obtained through therapeutic bleeding may be used for homologous transfusion if the unit is deemed suitable by the director of the blood bank. If it is to be used, the recipient's physician must agree to using the blood for his or her patient and a record should be kept of the agreement. The unit is then labeled and processed in the usual manner. The label must indicate that the blood is the result of a therapeutic bleed and include the patient's diagnosis. If the unit is not suitable for transfusion, the entire unit is disposed of in the usual manner of contaminated waste.

## PRIORITY LISTS

In the course of a day's work at a busy hospital or clinic, a phlebotomist may have to make decisions about the order in which blood work is obtained. Priorities must be set and adhered to whether they concern the order in which certain blood tests are drawn on a particular patient or which patients are to be drawn first among a group. If these distinctions are not made properly, test results can be affected and interpretation of the results may be very difficult.

## Patient Priorities

*Timed Specimens.* Whenever a test is ordered to be drawn at a particular time, it is the responsibility of the phlebotomist to see that blood is drawn as near to the requested time as is possible. The most common requests for timed specimens are glucose levels, drawn two hours after a meal. (Refer back to the section in this chapter on 2-hour post-prandial specimens.) The glucose value in the blood is constantly changing and it is most important that the blood not be drawn too early to give falsely elevated results, or too late to give a falsely normal result.

Other timed specimens may be for peak and trough levels of certain drugs. Often patients on drug therapy must be monitored to check if effective therapeutic levels are being given. If the trough level is too high, the drug may be discontinued for a period until the blood drug level returns to lower and safer levels. Again, the timing of the blood drawn on these patients can be critical and must be drawn as close as possible to the time ordered. If a time delay is unavoidable, the actual time of the collection must be indicated on the requisition form.

Certain natural hormone levels, such as cortisol, rise and fall with the time of the day. A sample of blood taken at 8:00 AM shows the highest value for cortisol during the day. A sample taken at 8:00 PM is usually approximately two-thirds of the morning sample. Therefore if a phlebotomist has difficulty obtaining a blood specimen on a patient at 8:00 AM, someone else should try as soon as possible afterwards, or the test may be cancelled until the following day at the discretion of the attending physician. Obtaining a specimen for cortisol at noon may give the doctor little information upon which to base his or her treatment.

*Fasting Specimens.* When a phlebotomist works at an institution that treats inpatients, care should be taken that the patient is not unduly inconvenienced by an order for fasting blood tests. The phlebotomist should arrange the order that he or she collects blood from neighboring patients such that a patient's meal is not kept waiting because his or her blood has not been drawn yet. Fasting levels of glucose, cholesterol, and triglycerides can be very important in diagnosis of patients and monitoring their progress during the hospital stay. If a patient is found not be fasting when the phlebotomist reaches him or her, the phlebotomist should consult with the physician to determine if a nonfasting level will be of any benefit. The slip should then indicate that the patient is nonfasting.

*"STAT" Specimen.* The term "STAT," which means, literally, immediately, has come to indicate a patient whose condition suddenly may become very critical and must be treated or responded to "STAT." When blood work is ordered "STAT," it generally means that a specimen should be

drawn and analyzed *immediately* in order to properly handle a critical patient. This requires an immediate response and effective technique from the phlebotomy team and constant availability of personnel for "STAT" blood collections. The phlebotomist should not only draw the blood quickly and properly, but should insure its timely delivery to the laboratory for "STAT" analysis. However, regardless of the physical state of the patient, the phlebotomist must adhere to the proper procedure for obtaining the best possible specimen from the patient. No shortcuts can be allowed in spite of the emergency situation that may be in progress. The phlebotomist has a responsibility to the patient to obtain a properly labeled, correct specimen for the test that is ordered. Anything less than that may lose precious time for the patient being treated while another specimen is being collected.

## Test Collection Priorities

Very often, multiple blood assays are ordered on patients. Whether the phlebotomist chooses to use a multiple-draw evacuated tube collection system or a plastic syringe, there are certain guidelines for delivery of blood into the proper collection tubes.

*Evacuated Tube Collection System.* Whenever coagulation studies are ordered, at least one other tube of blood should be drawn before the coagulation test specimen. This diminishes contamination with tissue fluids which may initiate the clotting sequence. Any tube that has an anticoagulant in it should be drawn last so that it can be mixed as soon after collection as possible. Care should be taken that the anticoagulant present in the tube does not come into contact with the multisample needle when changing tubes as some may be carried into the next tube and cause erroneous test results. For example, it is recommended that blood for serum iron be drawn *before* other specimens collected in tubes with chelating anticoagulants (e.g., EDTA) to avoid interference in testing the serum iron level. Generally, if the tube is held horizontally or slightly down during blood collection, transfer of anticoagulants from tube to tube will be minimal (Fig. 5-7).

*Syringe Collection.* When a phlebotomist chooses to use a syringe, the order of delivery of blood to the tubes changes considerably. If coagulation studies are ordered, the blood should be delivered to the sodium citrate tube first and mixed; next, blood should be delivered to any other anticoagulated tube and mixed. Finally, tubes without anticoagulant may be filled from the syringe. If a large volume of blood (at least 20 ml) has been drawn and there is a possibility that part of the blood may be clotted, the needle should be removed from the hub of the syringe, the stopper removed from the tube and the blood expelled into the tube along the side.

# Evacuated tube method

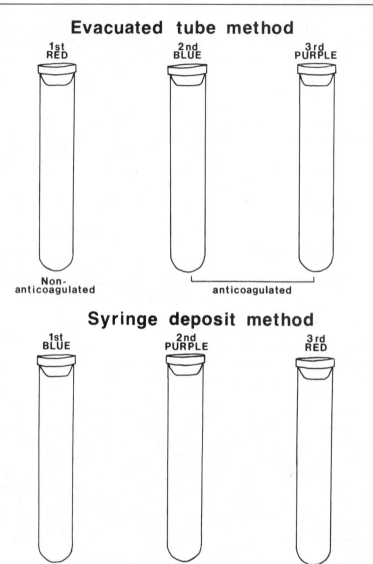

1st
RED

2nd
BLUE

3rd
PURPLE

Non-
anticoagulated

anticoagulated

# Syringe deposit method

1st
BLUE

2nd
PURPLE

3rd
RED

anticoagulated

Non-
anticoagulated

**Figure 5-7.** Order of draw.

When blood cultures are ordered, the procedure should be followed as previously described in the section on Blood Culture Collection. The blood should be delivered first aseptically into the culture bottle(s), then to the anticoagulated tubes, and finally to the tubes without anticoagulant.

The blood should always be delivered gently to the tubes to avoid hemolyzing the cells. This is done by directing the flow from the needle or the syringe hub along the side of the tube without foaming or extra pressure on the plunger. Evacuated tubes fill themselves and therefore the blood does *not* need to be forcefully ejected from the syringe.

## THE EMERGENCY CENTER

The phlebotomist's role in an emergency center (emergency room, ER, and so on) may vary from state to state, city to city, and hospital to hospital. Local laws may prohibit unlicensed persons from starting an IV in one state whereas there may be no restrictions in a neighboring state. The limitations placed on an unlicensed person may vary considerably; therefore if a phlebotomist is to be involved in the Emergency Center, he or she should become familiar with the limitations and expectations at the health institution.

The atmosphere in an emergency center is very different from any other area of the hospital. Most emergency rooms are chronically filled with people in pain, ranging from relatively minor injuries or illnesses to major, traumatic injuries. In addition to those who have come to the Emergency Center for immediate treatment of acute injuries or illness, there are those who have no regular physician and use the local emergency center for treatment of chronic illnesses such as coughs and colds. Family members often accompany the patients and may be highly emotional and vocal about their concern for loved ones.

This range of patients and families with varying needs, demanding attention from the limited staff, can create a highly charged atmosphere. Most Emergency Centers have a central reception area that prioritizes the patients as they come in. It is often referred to as a triage area. Those who need immediate attention are seen first and those whose conditions are more stable are seen later. However, even when the patients are prioritized according to their illnesses, the routine can be assaulted if a trauma patient arrives by ambulance and requires immediate life-saving measures. Although the triage desk may attempt to put order and stability in the Emergency Center workflow, medical emergencies and critically ill or injured patients are unavoidable and must be handled professionally. It is easy to see that the Emergency Center is an unpredictable setting. Although guidelines are placed on the flow of patients, the unexpected can occur at any moment.

Recognizing that the Emergency Center setting is a stressful one, the phlebotomist has two very important responsibilities. First, he or she must be completely familiar with all of the equipment and well-versed in all blood collecting procedures. If called upon to collect "STAT" blood specimens from a critically injured person about to go to surgery, the phlebotomist must respond quickly, and successfully obtain the correct specimen in the right volume. There may not be enough time to recollect the specimen if the first one is unsuitable. Only experienced phlebotomists should accept positions in the Emergency Center, where skills must be well-mastered and automatic. The second responsibility is to follow directions quickly and correctly. In a critical situation, it is vital that the phlebotomist follow the orders exactly and not require extensive time consuming directions. An experienced, confident, mature phlebotomist is best suited to the unpredictable emergency environment.

Another factor present in the Emergency Center, which may cause a great deal of stress in some persons, is the sight and sound of traumatically injured patients in pain. Profuse bleeding, disfigurement, moaning and groaning are common occurrences in this setting. It is wise for phlebotomists to be aware of their reactions to critically injured patients. If they find it too stressful, they should opt for work on the general floors of the hospital or in a clinic setting where the sights and sounds are more predictable and controlled. The phlebotomist who works in an Emergency Center must learn to do his or her job with single-mindedness and ignore anything that may distract from obtaining high quality samples with speed and accuracy.

Obviously in such a stress-charged atmosphere, tension runs high and minor personality conflicts occur more readily than in other more routine surroundings. The phlebotomist, like all Emergency Center personnel, must learn to resolve and quickly dismiss irritations and losses of temper that may otherwise interfere with the delivery of good emergency medical care. A mature, responsible person can best cope with the Emergency Center environment.

Emergency medicine is not for everyone; some can work in that environment for only a limited amount of time; others would work nowhere else. The excitement of being part of a team of professionals who routinely provide life-saving treatment to critically injured victims has an attraction that cannot be easily duplicated in any other area of patient care. Phlebotomists must choose the environment that is best suited to their temperament and where they can best deliver quality patient care.

## STUDY QUESTIONS

1. Why should the thumb not be used for palpating arteries in an arterial puncture?
2. Describe the preparation for an arterial puncture.
3. Why is the Ivy method for bleeding time the method of choice over the Duke method?
4. Describe the technique for properly preparing a site for a blood culture sample.

5. What is the purpose of skin testing?
6. What instructions should be given to a patient who is about to undergo a glucose tolerance test?
7. What role can a phlebotomist play in epinephrine or glucagon tolerance tests?
8. What is the sweat chloride test used for?
9. List the parts of the physical examination for donor acceptability.
10. What is the proper amount of blood taken from a donor to make one unit of blood?
11. Explain the purpose of therapeutic phlebotomy.
12. Name three ways in which blood specimens are ordered that influence the sequence in which the phlebotomist collects blood from patients.
13. Describe the order in which tests are drawn on a patient when using a syringe.
14. What are two important responsibilities that the phlebotomist has in an emergency room?

# REFERENCES

1. "Sweat Chloride by Iontophoresis" procedure used in Special Chemistry section of the Department of Pathology and Laboratory Medicine, Hermann Hospital, Houston, Texas. Method developed by Karen Kumor, M.D., 1981.
2. American Association of Blood Banking Technical Manual: Washington, D.C., 1981.
3. Bauer JD: Clinical Laboratory Methods. St. Louis, C.V. Mosby, 1982.
4. Lennette E, Spaulding E, Truant J: Manual of Clinical Microbiology. Washington, D.C., American Society for Microbiology, 1976.
5. Henry J: Clinical Diagnosis and Management by Laboratory Methods. Philadelphia, W.B. Saunders, 1979.

# CHAPTER 6

# Infection Control and Equipment Safety in Patients' Rooms

Kathleen Becan-McBride and Diana Garza

## INTRODUCTION TO INFECTION CONTROL

The condition in which the body is invaded with pathogenic bacteria, fungi, viruses, and/or parasites is called infection. Nosocomial infections are those which are acquired after admission to a health-care facility, including hospitals, clinics, nursing homes, and psychiatric institutions. Approximately 5 percent of hospitalized patients in the United States acquire nosocomial infections.[1] These infections are often harmful to the patient and costly to both patients and insurers. Each year millions of dollars are spent on nosocomial infections. In an attempt to control them, "infection control programs" have been developed. Based on guidelines established by the Center for Disease Control (CDC), the Joint Commission for Accreditation of Hospitals (JCAH), and state regulatory agencies, each health-care institution is responsible for developing and implementing an infection control program. These programs usually address the issues of surveillance, reporting, isolation procedures, education, and the investigation of epidemics, within the health-care institution. An infection control nurse or practitioner usually works closely with or in the clinical microbiology laboratory and communicates with personnel on the hospital ward to make the necessary assessments.

## Surveillance

In most health-care institutions, the infection control program monitors and collects data on several specific populations such as: (1) patients at a high risk of infection, (2) patients with already acquired infections, (3) personnel or patients accidentally exposed to communicable disease, contaminated equipment, or hazardous reagents, and (4) patients in certain areas of the hospital or in certain rooms. It is helpful to the phlebotomist to be aware of these special circumstances for two reasons. First, the phlebotomist can take the necessary precautions to avoid infecting him or herself or the patient. Second, the phlebotomist can mentally prepare him or herself to deal in a professional and humanistic manner with these special patients. Because each hospital has its own infection control programs and/or policy manual, it behooves the phlebotomist to read and familiarize him or herself with it.

Infection control surveillance also involves classification of infections according to prevalence rates. One example of a report depicting the prevalence of nosocomial infections is represented in Figure 6-1. Each of these infections can be transmitted in a variety of ways. The phlebotomist should realize that he or she can be a potential recipient or transmitter of infectious agents. Table 6-1 lists causative agents for nosocomial infections.

Infection control programs monitor employee health programs. A primary objective of both programs is to minimize the risk of infection or hazardous circumstances for employees and patients. Most employees are screened for the following diseases prior to working: measles, mumps, tuberculosis, hepatitis, diarrheal disease, syphilis, and skin diseases. Immunization for a variety of diseases is often made available initially and throughout employment, free of charge. Often, the hospital stipulates policies for employees with specific infections or who have been exposed to certain infections as in Table 6-2.

For the employee's protection, many types of warning labels are used. Among these are color-coded isolation signs and radiation hazard signs. Radiation signs may be posted on the hospital door of patients treated with radioactive isotopes. Generally speaking, a short period of contact with these patients would not be significant; however, the College of American Pathologists (CAP) recommends that pregnant employees avoid contact with these patients.[2]

## Modes of Transmission

Nosocomial infections result when the "chain of infection" is complete. The three components which make up the chain are source, means of transmission, and susceptible host.[1] In a normal environment, relatively few things are sterile, therefore, sources include a wide range of things. Inanimate objects, as well as people, are colonized with a variety of microorganisms, many of which help carry out normal bodily functions. Some of these

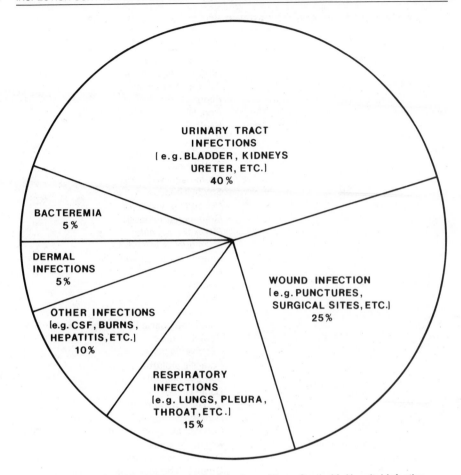

**Figure 6-1.** Prevalence of nosocomial infections. *(From Castle M: Hospital Infection and Control: Principles and Practice. New York, John Wiley and Sons, with permission.)*

microorganisms, however, are more pathogenic than others. For example, relatively few *Shigella* organisms need to be ingested for a diarrheal infection to occur. However, with *Salmonella,* large numbers of organisms need to be ingested before acquiring symptoms. On the other hand, numerous anaerobic and aerobic bacteria must be present in the gastrointestinal tract for normal metabolism to occur.

Regarding the sources of nosocomial infections, infection control practitioners must consider amount of contamination, viability of the infectious agent, virulence of the agent, length of time from contamination to contact, and how the agent was transmitted from the source. Sources of nosocomial infection can be hospital personnel, other patients, and visitors, and medi-

**TABLE 6-1. PATHOGENIC AGENTS CAUSING NOSOCOMIAL INFECTIONS**

| Body Areas or Hospital Areas | Commonly Identified Pathogenic Agents |
| --- | --- |
| Blood and cerebrospinal fluid | Any microorganisms |
| Burn unit | All gram-negative bacilli |
| | Gram-positive rods |
| | Fungi |
| Dialysis unit | Hepatitis and other viruses |
| | Bacteria |
| | Fungi |
| Ear | *Pseudomonas aeruginosa* |
| | *Streptococcus pneumoniae* |
| | Gram-negative bacilli |
| Eye | *Staphylococcus aureus* |
| | *Neisseria gonorrheae* |
| | Gram-negative bacilli |
| | *Moraxella lacunata* |
| | *Haemophilus influenzae* |
| | *Streptococcus pneumoniae* |
| | *Pseudomona aeruginosa* |
| Gastrointestinal tract | *Salmonella* sp. |
| | *Shigella* sp. |
| | *Yersenia enterocoliticus* |
| | Enteropathogenic *Escherichia coli* |
| | *Vibrio cholerae* |
| | *Campylobacter* sp. |
| | Parasitic protozoans |
| | *Candida albicans* |
| | Some viruses |
| Genital tract | *Neisseria gonorrheae* |
| | *Hemophilus vaginalis* |
| | *Candida albicans* (yeast) |
| Intensive care or postoperative unit | Any microorganisms |
| Nursery unit | *Staphylococcus aureus* |
| | Group B *Streptococcus* |
| | *Escherichia coli* |
| | *Streptococcus pneumoniae* |
| | Other gram-negative bacilli |
| | Viruses |
| Respiratory tract | *Streptococcus pyogenes* |
| | *Corynebacterium diphtheriae* |
| | *Bordatella pertussis* |
| | *Staphylococcus epidermidis* |
| | *Staphylococcus aureus* |
| | *Streptococcus pneumoniae* |
| | *Hemophilus influenzae* |
| | Any gram-negative bacilli |
| | Fungi |
| | Certain viruses |

*(continued)*

**TABLE 6-1.** *Continued*

| Body Areas or Hospital Areas | Commonly Identified Pathogenic Agents |
|---|---|
| Skin | *Staphylococcus aureus* |
| | *Streptococcus pyogenes* |
| | *Candida albicans* |
| | Smallpox |
| | Herpes virus |
| | Enterovirus |
| | Measles |
| Urinary tract | Any microorganism in sufficient numbers |
| Wounds and abscesses | Any microorganisms |

cal instruments, such as contaminated needles, intravenous catheters, Foley catheters, cardiac catheters, bronchoscopes, respiratory therapy equipment, and medical reagents (intravenous fluids and saline).

Human hands provide a warm moist environment for microorganisms. Therefore, a physician, phlebotomist, or nurse can transmit organisms from themselves or an infected patient to another potential host. Uniforms or other clothing, which have had contact with infectious agents, and are then used with other patients, are potential sources of infection. Medical instruments that come into contact with open wounds, mucous membranes, or organs present a possible source of infection. For example, an instrument, such as a fiberoptic bronchoscope, may be used repeatedly only if thoroughly decontaminated between patient use. Otherwise, it may be implicated in transmitting bacterial pneumonia. Many other pieces of invasive equipment are potential transmitters unless adequately sterilized. Some equipment can become contaminated with bacteria, yet is less likely to cause infection. As an example, tourniquets come in contact with intact skin, but are not likely to be a source of infection.

The next step in the link involves transmission from the source to the next host. Pathogenic agents may be transmitted by direct contact, via air, by medical instruments or other objects, or other vectors. Direct contact involves close or intimate contact with an infected person. For example, some patients acquire staphylococcal infections, chicken pox, hepatitis, or diarrhea after touching other infected individuals. During contact, the infective microorganism is rubbed off one person onto another. Handwashing is the best means of preventing infections by this route.

Microscopic airborne droplets may carry infectious agents, such as the causative agent of tuberculosis and Legionnaire's disease. Droplets may become airborne in the following instances: when an individual coughs or sneezes, when linens are shaken, when dust is stirred by sweeping, or when ventilation is not adequate. Means of prevention are wearing a mask, isolating specific patients, and good ventilation.

## TABLE 6-2. EMPLOYEE INFECTIONS OR SPECIAL CIRCUMSTANCES

| Disease | Work Status | Duration of Work or Work Limitations |
|---|---|---|
| Draining abscess, boils, and so forth | Off | Until drainage stops, if employee has patient contact |
| Chickenpox (varicella) | Off | For seven days after eruption first appears in normal host, provided lesions are dry when they return |
| Diarrhea Shigella Salmonella | Variable | Individual, depending on extent of symptoms, cultures, and evaluation by Personnel Health Service |
| Gonorrhea | May work | |
| Hepatitis A | Off | Must bring note from private physician upon return |
| Hepatitis B | Off | Must bring note from private physician upon return |
| Herpes simplex | May work | Evaluation by Personnel Health Service, depending on work area |
| Herpes zoster | No patient contact | If able to work, may do so |
| Influenza and URI | Variable | Evaluation by Personnel Health Service, depending on work area |
| Impetigo | Off | No patient contact until crusts are gone |
| German measles (rubella) | Off | Until rash is cleared (minimum of 5 days) |
| Measles | Off | Until rash is cleared (minimum of 4 days) |
| Mononucleosis | Off | At discretion of private physician |
| Positive PPD conversion | May work | Evaluation and follow-up by Personnel Health Service |
| Pregnancy (1st or 2nd trimester) | May work | Avoid patient contact with patients having viral or rickettsial infections or those being treated with radioactive material |
| Pregnancy (3rd trimester) | May work | Avoid contact with patients in any type of isolation |
| Active TB | Off | Until under treatment and smears are negative for 2 weeks |
| Scabies | Off until treated | |
| Strep throat (group A) | Off | May work after being placed on appropriate antibiotic and/or symptom free |

Sample guideline for employees with infections, their work status, and when they can return to work. (Adapted from Castle M: Hospital Infection Control Principles and Practice. New York, John Wiley & Sons, 1980, with permission.)

Invasive medical instruments, as well as other inanimate objects, may expose a susceptible patient to pathogenic agents. Instruments, such as tourniquets and catheters, should be changed after use or decontaminated. Needles should be disposed of after each use. Other objects, such as toys in the pediatric areas, common toilets and sinks, linens, and water fountains are all potential modes of transmission. Preventing these transmission modes can be accomplished by isolation techniques, utilization of sterile technique for injections or venipuncture, wearing gloves during equipment handling, and restricting use of common toys or facilities.

Many insects (mosquitos, ticks, fleas, mites) and rodents act as vectors in transmitting infectious diseases such as plague, rabies, and malaria. Patients may be exposed to them in unsanitary conditions or in areas where the diseases are prevalent.

The third area in the infectious chain is the susceptible host. Factors that affect host susceptibility are age, drugs, degree and nature of the illness, and status of the host immune system. The progress of the patient in the hospital greatly affects his or her chances of acquiring an infection. Underlying diseases, such as diabetes, immune deficiency syndrome, cancer, and therapeutic measures (chemotherapy, radiation therapy, antibiotics), all change the status of the body making it a potential host for infection.

Infection control programs aim at breaking the infection chain at one or more spots, as shown in Figure 6-2. Handwashing procedures for sterile techniques, proper waste disposal, appropriate laundry services, and housekeeping are ways of controlling the sources. Isolation techniques,

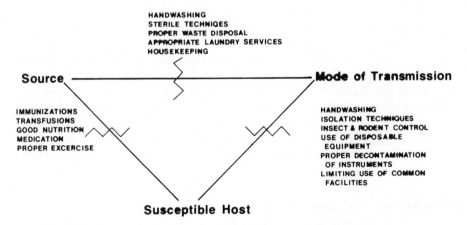

**Figure 6-2.** The chain of nosocomial infection can be interrupted by infection control procedures.

control of insects and rodents, use of disposable equipment and supplies help interrupt the modes of transmission. Host susceptibility is controlled by speeding the patient's recovery. Immunization, transfusions, nutrition, medication, and exercise all help the patient to regain his or her health.


## ISOLATION PROCEDURES

Isolation procedures, methods of removing diseased individuals from society, date back to antiquity. Although the supplies and methods have been updated, the fear of being contaminated and the stigma associated with a patient in isolation are still present. The psychologic affects of being a patient in isolation are profound. The phlebotomist should make an effort to reduce the anxiety of these patients by communicating in a calm, professional, and reassuring manner.

Isolation procedures are established in varying degrees. They range from sterile rooms or wards to isolation procedures for one disease only. However, in general, isolation techniques are divided into two types, procedures for patients with communicable diseases and procedures for patients who are extremely susceptible to infections.[1]

Most hospitals have special color-coded posters or signs on the patient's door indicating which type of isolation procedures is to be employed. The types and an actual procedure are listed below and shown in Figure 6-3 and Table 6-3.


### Strict or Complete Isolation

Strict or complete isolation is required for patients with contagious diseases, i.e., diseases which may be transmitted by direct contact, and via the air. Examples include anthrax, rabies, smallpox, measles, chickenpox, plague, diphtheria, streptococcal, and staphylococcal pneumonia. The patients are housed in private rooms with doors closed and all articles in the room should be handled as if they were contaminated. Patients are usually restricted to their rooms. If they must be moved, they should be appropriately covered. Personnel entering these rooms must wear gowns, a mask, and gloves. Handwashing is critically important. All items taken into the room must be left there in the appropriate location. (Refer to Table 6-3.)


### Respiratory Isolation

Respiratory isolation is required for patients with infections which may be transmitted through the air. Examples include tuberculosis, whooping cough, meningococcal meningitis, mumps, and measles. Patients are housed in private rooms with doors closed. Anyone entering the room

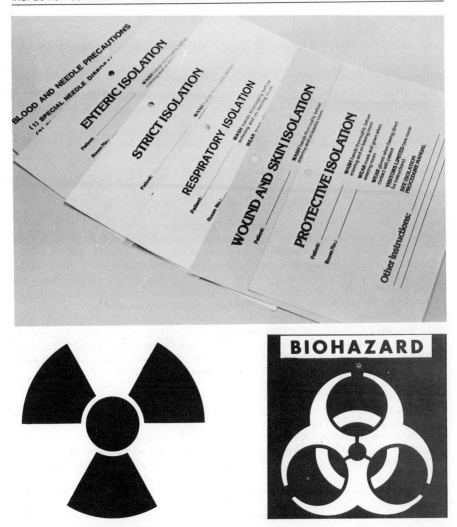

**Figure 6-3.** Isolation systems and warning signs.

must wear a mask, as should the patient if he or she is moved. All contaminated supplies should be disposed of in the patient's room.

### Enteric Isolation

Enteric isolation is required for patients with infections which are transmitted by ingestion of the pathogen. Examples include diarrheal diseases, such as *Salmonella, Shigella, E. coli, Yersinia, Staphylococcus, Campylobacter, Vibrio,* amebic dysentery, and other parasitic infections. Ideally, patients should be

## TABLE 6-3. ISOLATION TECHNIQUES FOR LABORATORY PERSONNEL

### Principle

Isolation techniques must be practiced by laboratory personnel when collecting specimens from infectious patients. This helps prevent the transmission of the disease to the laboratorian and to other patients via the technologist.

### Procedure

1. A sign posted on the door of an isolation room tells the technologist the type of isolation and to what extent the isolation procedures must be followed. The types of isolation are as follows:
   a. Complete: anthrax, rabies, smallpox, measles, chickenpox.
   b. Respiratory: tuberculosis, whooping cough, meningococcal meningitis, mumps, rubeola.
   c. Protective (reverse): immunosuppressed or burn patients.
   d. Wound and skin: postoperative.
   e. Enteric: hepatitis, *Salmonella, Shigella,* typhoid fever. Should also have "Needle and Blood Precautions" sign on the door.
2. Check with the nursing station to find out the diagnosis. Tell staff that you will ring for someone to receive the specimens at the doorway after you have drawn them.
3. Except for protective isolation, any equipment taken into the room must be left there. Make sure a Vacutainer adapter and tourniquet are in the room before entering. Protective isolation rooms should have an adapter and a tourniquet already in the room.
4. Isolation rooms have either an anteroom in which isolation equipment is kept or a cart outside the door for the same purpose.
5. Place a mask over nose and mouth. Tie both ties comfortably around head.
6. Put on a sterile gown, touching only the insides. Make sure the back is completely covered, and tie the belt. Pull the sleeves all the way down.
7. Put on disposable gloves, trying not to contaminate the palm with hands. Wash before entering a protective isolation room, wash your hands thoroughly before putting on sterile disposable gloves. Pull the gloves up over the sleeves of the gown.
8. Take only the needed equipment into the room.
9. Check the patient's armband and draw the specimen.
10. Dispose of the Vacutainer needle in the dirty needle box in the room. Throw the cotton swab and any gauze flats in the trash.
11. Turn on the call button for a member of the nursing staff to receive the specimens in an isolation bag at the door. Before placing tube in isolation bag, wipe the outside of the tubes with a paper towel moistened with cold water to remove any blood that may be on the outside of the tube.
12. Wash your gloved hands in the patient's room. Dry your hands and turn off the faucet with a paper towel.
13. Remove your face mask, touching only the strings.
14. Remove your gown by touching only the inside. Fold it with the contaminated side on the inside, and discard it.
15. Remove first glove.
16. Remove your second glove by sliding the pointer finger of the opposite hand between the glove and your hand. Discard the gloves.
17. Wash your hands again, using a paper towel to turn off the faucet.
18. Leave unit. Place clean paper towel over doorknob and open door. Hold door open with foot and discard paper towel in wastebasket beside door. Place tubes of blood in isolation container for return to laboratory.
19. Wash your hands at the nursing station before going to the next patient's room.

### Quality Control

The only means of quality control is strict adherence to the procedure.

*(Adapted from the University of Texas Department of Pathology and Laboratory Medicine, Hermann Hospital, Houston, Texas, with permission.)*

housed in private rooms. Their bathroom facilities should *not* be used by hospital personnel, other patients, or visitors. People entering these rooms should wear gowns and gloves. All contaminated materials should be disposed of in the patient's room.

## Wound and Skin Isolation

Wound and skin isolation may be required after surgery or if a patient is admitted with a skin infection. Postoperative wounds, catheters, and intravenous may become infected and microorganisms can be transmitted to other patients by direct or indirect contact. Patients are generally restricted to their rooms and all entering people should wear gowns and gloves. When these patients are moved, procedures to prevent transmission should be utilized, i.e., covering the infected site.

## Isolation Procedures for Hepatitis

Hepatitis may be transmitted directly or indirectly by blood and/or feces. Both enteric and blood precautions should be employed. Anyone handling blood or blood products from a patient with hepatitis should be warned. Patients with hepatitis should be in private rooms. Gowns and gloves should be worn if one is to have direct contact with the patient (as in venipuncture). If the patient is an asymptomatic carrier of the hepatitis B antigen, he or she should still be in a private room, however, good handwashing techniques will suffice to prevent transmission. All specimens from patients with hepatitis should be marked with warning labels.

Most laboratories have specific policies regarding the handling and labeling of specimens with suspected or known hepatitis. Specimens containing hepatitis virus particles should be segregated and handled separately. When these specimens are collected, centrifuged, and then poured into aliquots for the various laboratory procedures, the phlebotomist should be extremely cautious and note the following:

1. All specimens that have a request slip for hepatitis B surface antigen or antibody testing (except blood from healthy blood donors);
2. All icteric (dark yellow) serum;
3. All specimens with known previous positive hepatitis B surface antigen or antibody test;
4. All specimens identified as potential hepatitis by a referring facility.

Once these specimens are identified as "potential hepatitis" specimens, they must be properly labeled with the "biohazard" or "suspected hepatitis" label when separated into aliquots as they were labeled when collected. CAP guidelines indicate that the "biohazard" or "suspected hepatitis" label must be attached throughout the transmission of the specimen in the laboratory.[3]

## Isolation for Hospital Outbreaks

Occasionally, outbreaks of particular infections occur in one or more hospital areas. For example, infection control surveillance may reveal that the nursery unit is having many cases of staphylococcal infection. The infection control staff may dictate the need for special precautions, isolation procedures, or screening employees for staphylococcal carriers in order to control the outbreak. Anyone entering or exiting these areas, including phlebotomists, should be made aware of special circumstances.

## Other Diseases Requiring Isolation

*AIDS.* Some patients may have less commonly recognized infectious diseases which hospital personnel need to be aware of. Recently, many cases of acquired immunodeficiency syndrome (AIDS) have been reported. Associated with the syndrome are a variety of bacterial, fungal, viral, and parasitic diseases such as shigellosis, candidiasis, cytomegalovirus, gonorrhea, amebiasis, giardiasis, pneumocystic pneumonia, cryptosporidiosis, histoplasmosis, and infection with *Mycobacterium avium-intracellulare*.[4] The CDC recommends special precautions in handling these patients and their specimens. They include the following suggestions:[5]

1. Extraordinary care must be taken to avoid accidental wounds from needles contaminated with potentially infectious blood specimens, to avoid contamination with potentially infectious blood specimens, and to avoid contact of skin abrasions with blood from AIDS patients.
2. Gloves should be worn when handling blood specimens from AIDS patients.
3. Gowns should be worn when clothing may be soiled with blood or other body fluids.
4. Hands must be washed after removing gown and gloves and before leaving the room of a known or suspected AIDS patient. Hands should also be washed thoroughly and immediately if they become contaminated with blood.
5. The blood specimens from an AIDS patient should be labeled with the biohazard label or "AIDS Precautions" label and segregated from other specimens. If the outside of the specimen container is visibly contaminated with blood or a blood spill occurs, it should be cleaned with a disinfectant such as a 1 to 10 dilution of 5.25 percent sodium hypochlorite (household bleach) with water. The specimens should be placed in a bag as described earlier.
6. Articles soiled with blood should be placed in a biohazard labeled bag and an "AIDS Precautions" label should also be placed on it. At discard, these items should be autoclaved separately and may then be disposed of in the usual manner.

7. Needles should not be bent after use, but should be disposed of in the needle disposal container. Needles should not be reinserted into their original sheaths before being discarded into the container because a needle injury may result. Disposable syringes and needles should be used.

8. When centrifuging the blood from AIDS patients, gloves should be worn to avoid skin contact with blood. Laboratory coats, or gowns, should be worn during this process and should be discarded appropriately before leaving the laboratory.

*Creutzfeldt-Jacob Disease.* Creutzfeldt-Jacob disease (CJD) is a slowly progressing, fatal, viral disease of the nervous system. It occurs in middle-aged patients of both sexes. The main symptoms are dementia, coma, and death. It occurs throughout the world and it is believed that about 200 deaths per year in the United States occur due to the virus. Cases have been reported in patients receiving corneal grafts and in those having contact with contaminated electroencephalographic electrodes. It is thought to be transmitted via any break in the skin.[6]

Strict isolation procedures are not warranted for patients with CJD, however, special precautions include the following:[6]

1. Venipuncture needles must be autoclaved prior to disposal.
2. Blood and cerebrospinal fluid should be handled in the same manner as the specimens with hepatitis warnings.
3. Iodine preparations should be used instead of alcohol to decontaminate skin surfaces of infected patients.
4. Thorough handwashing should be done before and after contact with infected patients or specimens. Scrubbing with a brush should be avoided so as not to break the skin.
5. If the phlebotomist accidentally punctures him or herself with a contaminated needle, the wound should be cleansed with an iodine or phenolic antiseptic.

## Protective or Reverse Isolation

Many patients are put in isolation because they are highly susceptible to infection and need to be protected from the external environment. Therefore, it is referred to as protective or reverse isolation. The patient does not necessarily have an infection but has a lowered resistance. In general, a private room and good handwashing techniques are sufficient but more serious precautions such as gowns, gloves, and masks may be used. Articles may be removed from the room and do not need to be double-bagged since these patients do not have infections. However, articles entering the room must be sterile or carefully decontaminated.

A few hospitals in the United States have large protective isolation facilities. Patients with combined immunodeficiencies need to live in environments that are completely sterile. All food and articles are sterilized prior to entering the patient's room. Some patients must live their entire lives in this protected environment.

Other areas where patients are at a high risk of infection are the nursery, burn units, postoperative or intensive care units, and dialysis units.

## Infection Control Procedures in a Nursery Unit

Newborn infants are easy candidates for infections of all sorts because their immune systems are not fully developed at birth. They may pick up pathogens from their mothers, other babies, or hospital personnel. The best way to minimize infection is to use an antiseptic for handwashing. Special clothing changed daily may be worn by nursery personnel and limited to that unit. It has been recommended that bibs be used and discarded after contact with each baby. Often times a baby is assigned only one nurse so as to limit the possibility of transmitting infection. Babies whose mothers have genital herpes must be isolated from other infants. Mothers with genital herpes must also be isolated. All individuals having contact with either the mothers or children must be gowned, gloved, and double-bagging procedures must be employed for disposal of contaminated articles in the patient's room.

## Infection Control in a Burn Unit

Patients with burns are also highly susceptible to infection. In some institutions, infection rates are lower due to the availability of a completely isolated environment for each patient. Each bed is surrounded by a plastic curtain containing sleeves. Hospital personnel use these sleeves when contacting the patient. All supplies and equipment are kept outside of the curtain.[1]

In hospitals lacking these facilities, burn patients are housed in private rooms. Gowning, gloving, double-bagging (as described later in this chapter), and strict handwashing procedures should be utilized. All articles in the room, as well as the room itself, should be disinfected or sterilized frequently.

## Infection Control in an Intensive Care and/or Postoperative Unit

Patients in intensive care units (ICU) are more critically ill and, by the nature of being there, are more susceptible to infections. In most hospitals, ICUs are open areas with numerous patients in one large room so as to be more easily monitored. Patients with known infections should be isolated according to the type of infection they have and strict handwashing policies are necessary in all ICUs.

Postoperative patients are susceptible to infection because surgical wounds or drains enable bacteria to gain easy access to deeper tissues. Here again, patients should be isolated and dealt with according to the type of infection acquired.

## Infection Control in a Dialysis Unit

Patients needing dialysis are most often immunosuppressed, making them a high risk group for contracting infection, especially hepatitis. Protective gowns and gloves may be worn on the unit and strict handwashing techniques should be employed. Specimens should be marked with appropriate labels if hepatitis is known to exist.

## Infection Control in the Clinical Laboratory

The clinical laboratory contributes to infection control programs in the following manner:

- maintenance of laboratory records for surveillance purposes;
- reporting of infectious agents, drug resistant microorganisms, and outbreaks; and
- evaluating the effectiveness of sterilization or decontamination procedures.

Laboratory personnel must be cautious because they often handle specimens with infectious agents. Laboratorians have higher incidence of hepatitis antigen, tuberculosis, tularemia, and Rocky Mountain spotted fever than other hospital personnel.[1] Many of these infections are acquired by aerosols, needlesticks, spills, mouth pipetting, and eating, drinking or smoking in the laboratory. These can be easily avoided or minimized by adhering to policies which prohibit mouth pipetting, eating, drinking, and smoking in the laboratory. Handwashing, protective clothing, surface decontamination, and careful disposal of needles are also useful procedures.

Phlebotomists are usually headquartered in the clinical laboratory. It should be remembered that quality of laboratory results is only as good as the specimen collected. If the specimen is contaminated or improperly collected, laboratory results reflect this and may be misleading. If sloppy techniques are used, the potential for mistakes and infection is greater.

Phlebotomists are partially, if not fully responsible for the specimen collected. This includes proper collection procedures and adherence to policies. Infection control policies are often time consuming and cumbersome, however, failure to follow the policies results in more severe consequences. Because phlebotomists perform skin and venipunctures on numerous patients daily, their direct patient contact is considerable. In one day, a phlebotomist may collect specimens from fifty or so patients. Imagine the potential of that single phlebotomist to spread infections to all those patients if inappropriate procedures are followed. Phlebotomists are also fairly mobile individuals, i.e., they often have to collect specimens on several floors or in various parts of the hospital. This increases the likelihood of spreading infections to these areas if infection control policies are not followed. Table 6-4 details the responsibilities of the phlebotomist with regard to infection control policies.

**TABLE 6-4. INFECTION CONTROL RESPONSIBILITIES OF THE PHLEBOTOMIST**

1. Maintaining good personal hygiene including wearing clean clothes, keeping hair clean and tied back if necessary, keeping nails clean, and washing hands frequently.
2. Maintaining good health by eating balanced meals in the designated areas, getting enough sleep and exercise.
3. Reporting personal illnesses to supervisors.
4. Become familiar with and observe all isolation policies.
5. Learn about the job-related aspects of infection control and share this information with others.
6. Caution all personnel working with known hazardous material. This can be done with proper warning labels.
7. Report violations of the policies.
8. Report potential candidates for infection control, e.g., patients who are jaundice.

(From Forrest General Hospital: Infection Control Program, Laboratory Section. Hattiesburg, Mississippi, 1981, with permission.[7])

## SPECIFIC ISOLATION TECHNIQUES

In most hospitals, all supplies required for isolation procedures are located in an area or cart just outside the patient's room. After washing hands, the appropriate garb may be put on just prior to entering the room. (Refer to Fig. 6-4.)

### Handwashing

Handwashing is the most important procedure in the prevention of disease transmission in hospitals. It should be the first and last step of any isolation procedure. Scrubbing for surgery requires a different procedure than washing hands for general patient care. For general purposes, handwashing usually removes potential pathogens, but not necessarily sterilizes the hands. Good technique involves soap, warm running water, and friction.[1] Soap removes oils that may hold bacteria to the skin. Many varieties of soap are available for general purposes. However, it is recommended that hospitals choose those that are mild, easy to use, and form a good lather. Warm running water washes away loosened debris and lathers the soap. Friction from rubbing one's hands together loosens and removes dead skin, oil, and microorganisms. One should thoroughly rub both sides of each hand and in between each finger. Hands should be rinsed in a downward position. After rinsing, the faucet should be turned off using paper towels so as to avoid reinoculation of microorganisms onto hands.

### Masking

After washing hands, a mask (if necessary) may be put over the nose and mouth. Often a small metal band on the mask can be shaped to fit one's nose. Two ties are usually made, first one around the upper portion of the head, and second, around the upper portion of the neck. Most masks become ineffective after prolonged usage (20 minutes).[1]

## Gowning

A sterile gown should be put on by touching only the inside surface of it. It should have long sleeves and be large and long enough to cover all clothing. They are generally made of cloth or paper. The back must be completely covered, the belt tied, and the sleeves pulled all the way to the wrists.

## Gloving

Clean disposable gloves may be used for most isolation procedures. The exception is with protective isolation where sterile, disposable gloves should be used. Gloves should be pulled over the ends of the gown sleeve. It is recommended that rings or other jewelry not be worn as they may puncture the glove during patient contact.

## Entering and Exiting the Room

Isolation bags for transporting specimens are often available. The bag may be turned halfway inside out and left near the door outside the room or someone may be available to hold the bag outside the door. Only the needed supplies should be taken into the room. Phlebotomy requisitions may be left outside the room on the isolation cart. If drawing a blood specimen, the phlebotomist may use a tourniquet in the room, or leave the one brought in. The specimen should be labeled at the bedside and the pen left in the room. Used needles, swabs, and so on should be put in appropriate containers inside the room. Any blood on the outside of the specimen container should be removed with a paper towel. While standing in the doorway, and touching only the inside of the isolation bag, the specimen should be placed inside the bag. Gloved hands should be washed in the room. The faucet may be turned off with a paper towel.

The mask, if used, can be removed by carefully untying the lower tie first then the upper one. Only the ends of the ties should be held. It should then be properly disposed of inside the room. In some cases, a special container for masks is placed just outside the room to avoid exposure of hospital personnel to airborne diseases while inside.

The gown is removed first by breaking the paper tie or untying the sash. It should be removed and folded with the contaminated side turned inside and with care not to touch one's uniform. One glove may be removed, and the second one can be slipped off by sliding the index finger of the ungloved hand between the glove and the hand.

Just before leaving the room, however, hands must be washed again, using a paper towel to turn off the faucet. A clean paper towel should be used to open the door. The door should be held open with one's feet and used paper towels discarded in the waste basket directly inside the patient's room. Once outside the room, the requisition forms may be checked again, placed carefully in the isolation bag and sealed. Care must be taken to avoid

**Figure 6-4.** Specific isolation techniques: handwashing, masking, gowning, gloving, and double bagging.

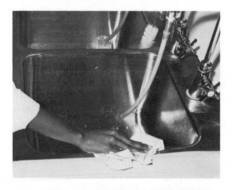
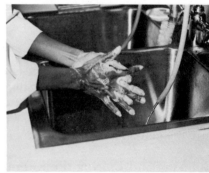
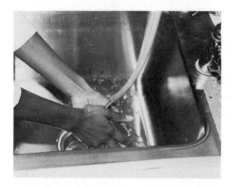

**A.** Good handwashing involves soap, warm running water, and thorough rubbing.

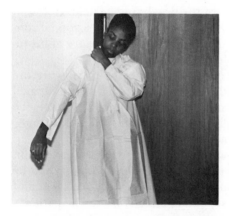
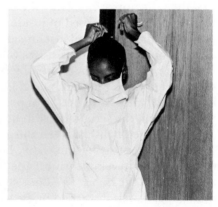

**B.** Gowns should be large enough to cover all clothing. Sleeves should be pulled down and back should be covered.

**C.** Masks should be tied in two places and fit comfortably.

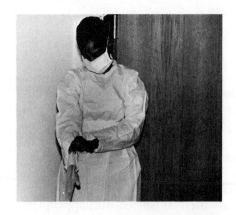

**D.** Gloves should be pulled over ends of gown sleeves. After specimen collection, removal of the gown should be from inside out.

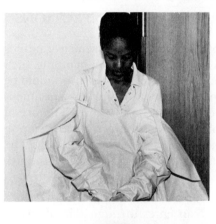

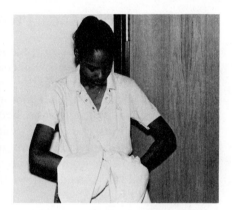

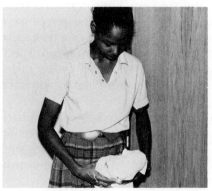

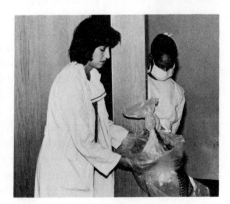

**E.** Double-bagging involves two individuals, one inside the room and one outside.

touching the inside of the bag holding the specimen. Personnel should wash hands again before proceeding with other duties.[8]

### Double-bagging

Trash, linens, and other articles in an isolation room must be removed by using the double-bagging procedure. Double-bagging involves putting contaminated material in one bag and sealing it inside the room. A different person should stand outside the doorway with another opened, clean, impermeable bag. The person standing outside the room should have the ends of the bag folded over the hands to shield them from possible contamination. The sealed bag from the room may then be placed inside the clean bag. The person outside the room can then fold over the edges, expel the air, and seal the outer bag. It should then be labeled with appropriate warnings.

## PREVENTION OF LABORATORY ACQUIRED INFECTIONS

As previously mentioned, the phlebotomist must be extremely cautious with biohazardous specimens. Policies and procedures for handling such specimens should be defined in the laboratory policy manual and should be reviewed periodically by the phlebotomist. Infections from these specimens may be spread in collection and handling by several routes. The actual occurrence of an infection from a biohazardous specimen depends upon the virulence of the infecting agent and the susceptibility of the host. The following are possible routes of infection from collected specimens, and, therefore should be considered when collecting or processing specimens for laboratory assays:

1. *Skin contact.* Virulent organisms can enter through skin abrasions and cuts or through conjunctiva of the eye. Thus, scratches from needles and broken glass must be avoided. If the phlebotomist has a cut or abrasion, he or she should wear a finger cot or protective adhesive tape to prevent possible inoculation from infectious specimens. The phlebotomist must avoid rubbing his or her eyes in order to prevent possible transmission of an infection from a biohazard specimen.

2. *Ingestion.* Failure to wash contaminated hands and subsequent handling of cigarettes, gum, food, or drinks can result in an infection from a biohazardous specimen. The phlebotomist must comply with the safety rules of the laboratory (see Chapter 9 on Safety) to prevent transmission of infections.

3. *Airborne.* As discussed in other sections, aerosols created from patients' specimens by careless splashing and/or centrifugation must be prevented by the phlebotomist and other laboratory personnel.

## SAMPLE HANDLING

The College of American Pathologists (CAP) Inspection and Accreditation Checklist states: "Laboratory infections have become a major laboratory hazard. Specimens from patients suspected or known to have hepatitis should be labeled in a distinct manner and handled and disposed of in a manner to minimize the hazard."[9] Each phlebotomist should thus carry plastic Ziploc bags and a small supply of biohazard labels (refer to Fig. 6-3) on his or her collecting tray. Specimens collected from "high risk" patients in enteric isolation, from known AIDS and known hepatitis patients should be labeled with a biohazard label at the time of collection. The blood identified as potential hepatitis is frequently labeled with a "Suspected Hepatitis" label. Those specimens from AIDS patients are sometimes identified with an "AIDS Precautions" label instead of biohazard label. The biohazardous specimen should be placed in a plastic bag and the request slip attached to the outside of the bag with a paper clip. If more than one biohazardous specimen is collected during a run, they may be placed in the same plastic bag and the request slips attached to the outside of the bag.[10]

It should be emphasized that no means of identifying all potentially hazardous specimens exists; therefore, care should be taken to avoid contact with all specimens. To alert laboratory collectors to potential biohazards, a list of known or suspected hepatitis and AIDS patients should be posted in the clinical laboratory or on the hospital floors.

### Infectious Aerosols

The phlebotomist should be aware that dangerous, infectious aerosols can be caused from popping stoppers off of the blood specimen vacuum tubes and centrifugation of the blood specimens.[11] Specimens from patients having hepatitis, AIDS, and other highly infectious diseases should be opened under a biologic safety hood or covered with a disinfectant pad at the time of opening. When opening the vacuum tubes, the caps should be twisted instead of popped.

Vacuum tubes should be inspected for cracks prior to centrifugation. Tubes with wet rims should be wiped dry prior to centrifugation. The centrifuge brake should not be applied to save time because braking can cause infectious aerosol formation. For blood specimens from "high risk," hepatitis, and AIDS patients, centrifuge trunnion cups with screw caps or equivalent apparatus should be used. The centrifuged infectious specimens must not be poured because of the potential hazards from aerosol formation. Instead, the contents should be transferred using a disposable pipet with rubber bulb or equivalent and gently transferring the contents down the wall of the aliquot tube(s).

## STERILE TECHNIQUES FOR PHLEBOTOMISTS

All hospital personnel should realize that bacteria and other microorganisms can be found everywhere. For example, human skin is covered with bacteria. Because of this fact, all hospital personnel should be responsible for cleanliness and maintaining sterility when handling instruments, catheters, intravenous supplies, or other devices that contact patients.

The phlebotomist has the responsibility of using sterile supplies for skin and venipuncture and antiseptics for patient preparation. Alcohol pads are often used to cleanse skin sites for venipuncture. Although rubbing with alcohol pads destroys most of the bacteria, it does not destroy all microorganisms. A special decontamination procedure is required to obtain a sterile site. Venipuncture for blood cultures requires this type of preparation, as discussed thoroughly in Chapter 5. It involves cleansing the site with surgical green soap for 2 minutes, removing the soap using a sterile alcohol pad, and applying an iodine solution in concentric circles beginning at the site and working outward. The iodine solution should be allowed to dry. In some hospitals, it is recommended that the tops of the blood culture bottles or tubes and the phlebotomist's finger used for palpation be sterilized in the same manner. (Refer to Chapter 5 for further details of the procedure.) Failure to use the proper technique may result in false positive blood cultures which are due to skin or needle contaminants.

New needles and most blood collection tubes are sterilized by the manufacturers. Once the covering of a needle or lancet has been removed, it should not touch anything until it punctures the skin. If it accidentally touches *anything* prior to the skin site, it must be appropriately discarded and replaced with a new one. If a needle is used for an unsuccessful venipuncture, it *must* be discarded and replaced with a new one before attempting another puncture.

Sterile techniques and isolation procedures may require sterile gloves. If such is the case, the phlebotomist must make sure that the package of gloves indicates that they are sterile. Some manufacturers produce gloves which are chemically clean but not necessarily sterile. Most sterile gloves come in various hand sizes. If gloves do not fit properly, they may interfere with the procedure.

### Disinfectants and Antiseptics

Disinfectants are chemical compounds used to remove or kill pathogenic microorganisms. Antiseptics are chemicals used to inhibit the growth and development of microorganisms but not necessarily kill them. Antiseptics may be used on human skin. Disinfectants are generally used on surfaces and instruments because they are too corrosive for direct use on skin. Table 6-5 lists some of the more common hospital disinfectants and antiseptics used.

**TABLE 6-5. COMMON HOSPITAL ANTISEPTICS AND DISINFECTANTS**

| Compound | Uses and Restrictions |
|---|---|
| *Alcohols* | |
| Ethyl | Antiseptic for skin |
| Isopropyl | Antiseptic for skin |
| *Chlorine* | |
| Chloramine | Disinfectant for wounds |
| Hypochlorite solutions | Disinfectant |
| *Ethylene oxide* | Disinfectant (toxic) |
| *Formaldehyde* | Disinfectant (noxious fumes) |
| *Glutaraldehyde* | Disinfectant (toxic) |
| *Hydrogen peroxide* | Antiseptic for skin |
| *Iodine* | |
| Tincture | Antiseptic for skin (can be irritating) |
| Iodophors | Antiseptic for skin (less stable) |
| *Mercury compounds* | Antiseptic for skin |
| *Phenolic compounds* | |
| 1–2% Phenols | Disinfectant |
| Chlorophenol | Disinfectant (toxic) |
| Hexachlorophene | Antiseptic for skin (used in surgery) |
| Chlorohexidine | Antiseptic for skin |
| Hexylresorcinol | Antiseptic for skin |
| *Quarternary ammonium compounds* | Antiseptic for skin (ingredient in many soaps) |

# EQUIPMENT AND SAFETY IN PATIENTS' ROOMS

As a member of the health-care team, the phlebotomist is responsible for the safety of the patient. All health-care professionals are responsible for patient safety from the time the patient enters the health-care setting until departure. As a matter of general patient safety, the phlebotomist should be aware of the following precautions in the patient's room:

1. Make certain that all specimen collection supplies, needles, and equipment are returned to the specimen collection tray after collection.
2. Check to see if the bedrails are up or down. Always place bedrails up before leaving the patient if they were up when entering the room.
3. Unusual odors should be reported to the nursing station because a pipe may be broken and leak gas or liquid.
4. Check for food or liquid spilled on the floor, urine spills, or IV leakage. Areas on which the patient and health-care professionals walk must be dry. They should be free of obstacles and slipping hazards. Thus, in case of spills, make certain that the area is cleaned and dried for the safety of the patient and hospital personnel.
5. To avoid a fire hazard, full ashtrays should be emptied in the toilet, but *never in the trash can.*

6. During blood collection, be very cautious not to touch an electrical instrument located adjacent to the patient's bed. If the instrument should malfunction, then the phlebotomist may ground the patient and as a result, a microshock would pass through the phlebotomist into the patient. A serious problem could result from this shock to a patient with an electrolyte imbalance or one who is wet with perspiration or other fluid. The needle inserted in the patient's arm could produce ventricular fibrillation and death if the patient has a pacemaker or an unstable heart ailment.

7. If the patient has an IV and the site is swollen and red in appearance, the IV needle is probably no longer in the vein and the IV solution is infiltrating into the surrounding tissues. Report this problem immediately to the nursing station because some chemicals in IV solutions are toxic to body tissue and gangrene could result due to infiltration. Also, if blood is backing up the IV line from the needle insertion to the IV drip container, the IV solution container is empty. Report this problem immediately.

8. If the patient is in unusual pain or unresponsive (see Chapter 9 on Emergency Procedures), notify the nursing station immediately.

## PATIENT SAFETY OUTSIDE THE PATIENTS' ROOMS

The phlebotomist should be aware of possible hazards to patients outside of the patients' rooms. As a matter of general safety practice, the phlebotomist should follow the following guidelines:

1. Because trays, carts, and ladders may be placed around a hallway corner, the phlebotomist should be careful about traveling too quickly from one room to another and around corners.

2. Items lying on the floor, such as flower petals, may cause someone to slip and should be reported for cleaning.

3. Avoid running in a hospital because patients and visitors may become alarmed and begin to run as well. Also, someone may be hurt if the phlebotomist runs into them (i.e., a cardiac patient walking in hall with inserted IV stand, another phlebotomist carrying specimen collection tray, and so forth).

## STUDY QUESTIONS

The following questions may have one or more answers.

1. Which of the following nosocomial infections is most prevalent?

a. dermal infections     c. respiratory tract infections

b. wound infections     d. urinary tract infections

**2.** Name the links in the infection control chain.

    **a.** poor isolation technique     **c.** source

    **b.** susceptible host          **d.** mode of transmission

**3.** What is (are) the primary function(s) of isolation procedures?

    **a.** Keep the hospital clean.     **c.** Protect the general

    **b.** Prevent transmission          public from disease.

       of communicable diseases.    **d.** Provide protective

                                 environments.

**3.** Phlebotomists are responsible for knowing procedures of which type(s) of isolation?

    **a.** strict              **d.** protective/reverse

    **b.** wound and skin    **e.** respiratory

    **c.** enteric

**5.** Which of the following precautions to avoid infectious aerosols is (are) true?

    **a.** To open a vacuum collection tube, pop the cap rather than twist it.

    **b.** Vacuum tubes should be inspected for cracks prior to centrifugation.

    **c.** The centrifuge brake can be applied to save time when centrifuging these specimens.

    **d.** It is best to pour the specimens into the required aliquots to avoid infectious aerosols.

**6.** Which of the following safety rules should be maintained in patient rooms?

    **a.** Full ashtrays should be emptied into the trash can to avoid a fire hazard.

    **b.** Unusual odors in the patient's room should be reported to the nursing station.

    **c.** Phlebotomists should not touch electrical instruments located adjacent to the patient's bed.

    **d.** If the patient has an IV and the site is swollen and reddish, this problem should be reported to the nursing station.

**7.** Which of the following precautions should be taken with patients who have or are suspected to have Acquired Immune Deficiency (AIDS)?

    **a.** Gloves should be worn when handling blood specimens from AIDS patients.

**b.** The blood specimen from an AIDS patient should be labeled with the biohazard label or "AIDS Precaution" label.

**c.** Articles soiled with blood should be placed in a biohazard labeled plastic bag and "AIDS Precautions" label should be placed on it.

**d.** Needles used to collect blood from AIDS patients should be bent after use and discarded.

## REFERENCES

1. Castle M: Hospital Infection Control, Principles and Practice. New York, John Wiley & Sons, 1980.
2. Valaske MJ: So You're Going to Collect a Blood Specimen. Skokie, Ill. College of American Pathologists, 1982.
3. Duckworth J: Clinical Laboratory Precautions Against Viral Hepatitis. Skokie, Ill., College of American Pathologists, October, 1976.
4. Pitlik SD, Fainstein V, Garza D, et al: Human cryptosporidiosis. Spectrum of disease: Report of six cases and review of the literature. Arch Intern Med 143:2269 – 2275, 1983.
5. Acquired Immune Deficiency Syndrome (AIDS): Precautions for Clinical and Laboratory Staff. Atlanta, GA, CDC: Center for Infectious Diseases, Office of Biosafety, Division of Safety, November, 1982.
6. Gajdusek C, Gibbs CJ, Asher DM, et al: Precautions in the medical care of, and in handling materials from, patients with transmissible virus dementia (Creutzfeldt-Jacobs Disease). N Engl J Med 297:1253 –1258, 1977.
7. Forrest General Hospital: Infection Control Program, Laboratory Section. P.O. Drawer 1897, Hattiesburg, Miss., 1981.
8. Hermann Hospital: Procedure Manual: Isolation Technique for Laboratory Personnel. Houston, Texas, Hermann Hospital, 1981.
9. College of American Pathologists: Commission of Inspection and Accreditation, Inspection Checklist Section III: Chemistry. Skokie, Ill., College of American Pathologists, March, 1979.
10. Lorimor K, Collins F: Monitoring Quality Control in the Clinical Laboratory in Textbook of Clinical Laboratory Supervision. New York, Appleton-Century-Crofts, 1982.
11. Stern E, Johnson J, Vesley D, et al: Aerosol production associated with clinical laboratory procedures. Am J Clin Path 62:591 –600, 1974.

# CHAPTER 7

# Communication and Specimen Transportation

Pamela Bollinger and Carrie Brailas

## PATIENT – PHYSICIAN – LABORATORY COMMUNICATION CYCLE

Communications, both written and verbal, are an integral part of all medical care. Because the major purpose of a clinical laboratory is the acquisition and determination of valid data by analytic procedures performed on patient specimens and the timely communication of those data to the physician, it is essential that a patient–physician–laboratory communication cycle be established to achieve this end. The number of persons and steps involved in this cycle varies greatly depending on the size of the institution and type of laboratory involved. With each additional step or person involved, however, another potential source of error or delay is introduced into the system. Therefore, it is the responsibility of the clinical laboratory to concern itself with all parts of the cycle rather than limit its attention solely to data acquisition. The phlebotomist is a vital link in this cycle and can serve to enhance communication between the patient, the laboratory, and the physician.

Various illustrations conceptualize this cycle pattern, ranging from a simplified version, as in Figure 7-1, to more complex representations as in Figures 7-2 and 7-3. Although these three illustrations are quite different, they all show that the clinical laboratory is intimately involved in extralaboratory activities in its effort to deliver effective services, and also that there is a constant overlapping or interaction between internal and exter-

158

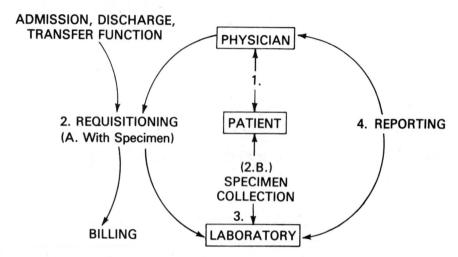

**Figure 7-1.** Communication functions are depicted in the patient – physician – laboratory communication cycle. *(From Henry J (ed): Clinical Diagnosis and Management by Laboratory Methods, WB Saunders Co, with permission.)*

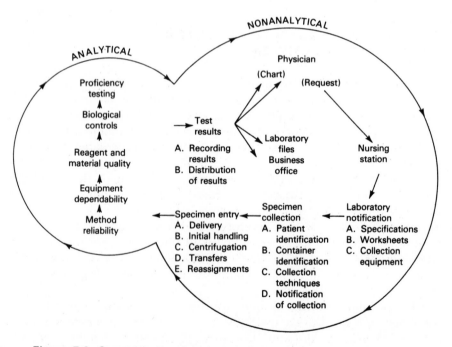

**Figure 7-2.** Communication functions are depicted in more detail in the patient – physician – laboratory communication cycle. *(From Shuffstall R, Hemmaplardh B: The Hospital Laboratory, CV Mosby Co, with permission.)*

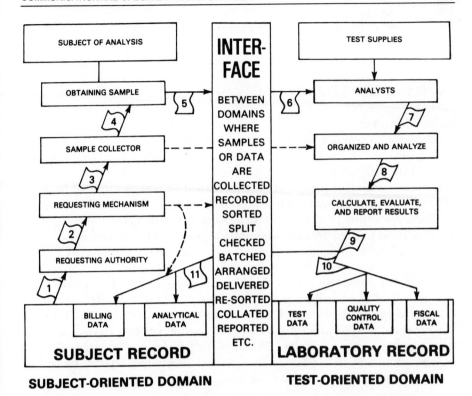

**Figure 7-3.** Communication functions may be very complex in nature. These functions are all vital to the efficiency of the patient – physician – laboratory communication cycle. *(From Inhorn S (ed): Quality Assurance Practices for Health Laboratories, American Public Health Association, with permission.)*

nal functions of the laboratory. This chapter addresses the importance of communication, both inside and outside the laboratory, as well as the various nonanalytic communication components of request specifications, test requisitioning, patient and specimen identification, specimen transport, reporting of results, and distribution of results; all of which are integral parts in the patient–physician–laboratory communication cycle.

Standard III of the College of American Pathologists (CAP), Standards for Accreditation of Medical Laboratories, 1974, states that, "channels of communication within the laboratory as well as with all other closely affiliated sections of services in the hospital and the medical staff shall be appropriate to the size and complexity of the organization."[1] In a relatively small laboratory, as in the case of a physician's office laboratory, the communication processes, both within the laboratory (intralaboratory) and with all others outside the laboratory (extralaboratory), are essentially the same. As the size of the institution increases, however, the requirements for both intralaboratory and extralaboratory communications are greatly expanded.

## INTRALABORATORY COMMUNICATIONS

### Policy Manual

Usually, each clinical laboratory has an administrative policy manual that can be consulted by all workers. The manual contains policies that are consistent with those of the larger organization (i.e., hospital, clinic). They are general in scope and particularly concerned with, but not limited to, such subjects as management authorizations, tables of organization, responsibilities, personnel practices, and professional protocol. As points of reference, written policies for the laboratory ensure consistency of intent, and save considerable time by removing the need to remake decisions. They are written in consultation with the clinical laboratory employees involved and reviewed for consistency with the institutional policies. The policies are generally approved and signed by the laboratory director. Because many changes occur in the clinical laboratory, the policies must be reviewed by the supervisory staff and updated at least annually with a signature and a date to document the review. When a staff technologist, technician, or phlebotomist accepts a position in a clinical laboratory section, he or she should become acquainted with the laboratory policies.[2]

### Procedure Manuals

Written procedures that provide information relevant to a given situation, event, or problem or protocol to be followed are usually made available to the clinical laboratory employees. Various types of written procedural manuals include the following.[2]

*Technical Procedures.* Technical procedures describe in detail the steps to be followed in the performance of specimen collection and each laboratory test. Usually, technical procedures are approved and signed by the supervisor of the section responsible for the performance of the particular laboratory test. The College of American Pathologists (CAP) requires technical procedures to be made available, on site at all times, to technical personnel who perform specimen collection and laboratory assays. The technical procedure format also includes normal range, clinical significance of results, quality control instructions, approval signatures, dates, method history, and references.

*Laboratory Administrative Procedures.* Laboratory administrative procedures pertain to administrative concerns. They are distributed to laboratory management and made available to all other relevant personnel. The following information is generally found in an administrative procedure manual:

- Technical procedure format
- Assignment of test code numbers to laboratory procedures
- Communication with physicians and other health-care professionals
- Time cards
- Attendance records
- Laboratory equipment identification and centralization of specification files
- Handling of samples for reference laboratory work
- Acceptable symbols, abbreviations, and units of measure
- Handling of laboratory charge tickets
- Purchase and repair requisitions
- Performance evaluation procedure
- Employee folders
- Distribution of laboratory documents
- Quality control procedures
- Safety procedures
- Loan of laboratory equipment
- Compensatory time off
- Employee accidents
- Laboratory libraries
- Disposal of capital equipment
- Disaster plan
- Consent to donate blood and urine specimens
- In-service records
- Clinical laboratory samples referred from outside sources
- Formal disciplinary action
- Hepatitis testing of laboratory personnel

*Safety Procedures.* Safety procedures should be distributed to all management and made known to all personnel. One book of safety procedures should be available in each laboratory section, including the specimen collection area.

*Quality Control Procedures.* Quality control procedures pertain to the conduct of diagnostic laboratory testing. One book of quality control procedures should be available in each laboratory section, including the specimen collection area.

Using well-written procedures in the clinical laboratory enhances the communication network by assuring continuity of methods; avoiding shortcuts; minimizing the chances of errors, specimen recollections and reruns; preventing expensive substitutions of reagents; and enhancing quality control, teaching, and safety. Overall, the procedures lead to more efficient data collection.

## Continuing Education

In addition to procedure manuals, ongoing laboratory in-service education programs help increase communication and efficiency in patient care. With the increasing complexity of laboratory medicine services, it is essential for phlebotomists to attend in-service education sessions. Phlebotomists are also encouraged to attend other appropriate educational programs within the institution and elsewhere. (Refer to Chapter 10 for information on planning educational programs.)

## Staff Meetings

Intralaboratory communications are improved when regularly scheduled staff meetings are held within each laboratory section, such as the specimen collection area. They are useful for discussing problems, new policies and procedures, and for planning. Decisions made in such meetings are usually conferred to all members of the laboratory by written memo, minutes of meetings, or by telephone contact in some cases.

## Memoranda

Effective communication through memoranda requires a concise, clear message written about one subject. This form of written communication should be written in a positive, courteous, and constructive manner. Memoranda provide a method for documenting conversations, decisions, agreements, and policies. They can be filed for future reference and reviewed before meetings. To avoid overstepping boundaries of authority, the phlebotomist should follow the hierarchical structure of the organization if he or she wishes to send memoranda or other written communications.[2]

## Other Modes of Intralaboratory Communications

Bulletin boards, posters, and clipboards are other suggestions for disseminating current information. One person from each laboratory should be responsible for periodically checking and changing poster information.

# EXTRALABORATORY COMMUNICATIONS

## Providing Information

Communication with other health-care professionals working outside of the laboratory is enhanced in a variety of ways. An information bulletin or "floor book" of laboratory services, made available at least in every patient unit, both inpatient and outpatient, is a handy reference. It contains a directory of the laboratory sections with listings of the key staff members, the location of the laboratory, telephone numbers, operating hours, instructions, and pertinent standard procedures of the laboratory. The methods used for collection of all specimens, and the proper identification, storage, preservation, and transportation mechanisms to be used are clearly specified. In addition, an alphabetical listing of all laboratory determinations, specimen requirements, special instructions, and normal values for each measurement are included (Figs. 7-4 and 7-5, and Table 9-1). The phlebotomist should be familiar with the floor book in order to answer questions related to the clinical laboratory specimen collections and procedures.

Periodic hospital and/or departmental newsletter or bulletins, circulated to all departments and medical staff, is another method of communicating information about new institutional and departmental services or policies. The phlebotomist should read these bulletins in order to learn more about the health-care institution and laboratory in which he or she works.

## Use of the Telephone

The telephone is the most frequently used method of two-way communication in any setting. Phlebotomists should be aware of the following procedures for operating it: how to transfer calls, putting someone on

| TEST # | PROCEDURE | SPECIMEN | REQUEST FORM | COLLECTED BY | INSTRUCTIONS |
|---|---|---|---|---|---|
| 131 | Carotene, Serum | Blood 10cc-R.T. | Special Test | Laboratory | To be collected by Laboratory and kept in dark. Performed by Reference Laboratory |
| 755 | Catecholamines | Urine 24-hr | Chem Urine II | Nurse | MUST be collected in rigid polyethylene container. Have Lab add conc. HCl before beginning collection. Keep cold. Deliver IMMEDIATELY |
| 203 | Catecholamine plasma | Blood 7cc-G.T. | Special Test | Laboratory | Collect on ice and bring IMMEDIATELY to Lab. Performed by Reference Laboratory |
| 300 | CBC (Complete Blood Count) | Blood 3cc-L.T. | Hematology I | Laboratory | |
| 340 | Cell Count, Miscellaneous Fluids | Fluids | Miscellaneous Fluids | Physician | MUST specify source |
| 100 | Chemical Survey (SMA 12/60), T. Protein Alb., Ca., I. Phos., Glu., BUN, Uric Acid, Creat., T. Bil., ALK. P'Tase, LDH, SGOT | Blood 10cc-R.G.T. | Chemistry I | Laboratory | Performed Sunday thru Friday |
| 145 | Chloride | Blood 7cc-R.T. | Chemistry I | Laboratory | |
| 146 | Chloride | CSF | Spinal Fluid | Physician | |
| 754 | Chloride | Urine | Urine Chemistry I | Nurse | |
| 150 | Cholesterol | Blood 10cc-R.G.T. | Chemistry III | Laboratory | Fasting specimen |

**Figure 7-4.** Excerpt from the laboratory bulletin of information listing all pertinent requirements regarding laboratory determinations. *(Courtesy of the University of Texas M.D. Anderson Hospital, Department of Laboratory Medicine.)*

NORMAL VALUES IN HEMATOLOGY

| TEST # | TEST NAME | NORMAL VALUES |
|---|---|---|
| 324 | White Blood Cell Count (WBC) | 4.0-11.0 K/μl |
| 321 | Red Blood Cell Count (RBC) | 4.50-6.00 M/μl (male) |
| | | 4.00-5.50 M/μl (female) |
| 365 | Hemoglobin | 14.0-18.0 g/dl (male) |
| | | 12.0-16.0 g/dl (female) |
| 360 | Hematocrit | 40.0-54.0% (male) |
| | | 37.0-47.0% (female) |
| | Indices | |
| 304 | MCV | 82-98 fl |
| 306 | MCH | 27.0-31.0 pg |
| 307 | MCHC | 31.0-36.0% |
| 327 | Platelet Count | 140-440 K/μl |
| 315 | Differential Count | |
| | Bands | 3-5% |
| | Neutrophils | 42-68% |
| | Lymphocytes | 24-44% |
| | Monocytes | 2-7% |
| | Eosinophils | 1-3% |
| | Basophils | 0-1% |
| | Absolute Granulocyte Count | 4,300 ± 1,520/μl |
| 318 | Eosinophil Count | Average of 200/μl |
| 355 | Erythrocyte Fragility | Initial hemolysis: 0.45-0.39% |
| | | Complete hemolysis: 0.33-0.30% |
| 375 | L.E. Cell Prep | Negative - no L.E. cells present |
| 330 | Reticulocyte Count | 0.5-1.5% |
| | Absolute Reticulocyte Count | 20,000-90,000/μl |
| 390 | Sedimentation Rate | 0-9 mm/hr (male) |
| | | 0-20 mm/hr (female) |
| 395 | Sickle Cell Test | Negative - no sickling detected |
| 350 | Spinal Fluid Cell Count | Up to 10 lymphocytes/μl |
| 380 | Alkaline Phosphatase, Leukocyte (total score) | 40-120 (male) |
| | | 40-225 (female) |
| 385 | Prothrombin Time (PT) | 10.2-12.6 seconds |
| 376 | Partial Thromboplastin Time (PTT) | 24.4-35.8 seconds |
| 398 | Fibrinogen | 200-400 mg/100 ml |
| 359 | Fibrin Degradation/Split Products | <10 μg/ml |
| 305 | Bleeding Time | 2.5-7.5 minutes |
| 332 | Sucrose Presumptive Test for PNH | Negative |
| 384 | Prothrombin Consumption Time | >20 seconds |
| 361 | Thrombin Time | 12.7-16.7 seconds |
| 354 | Reptilase Time | 14.6-19.8 seconds |
| 356 | Antithrombin III (AT III) | 80%-100% normal activity |

**Figure 7-5.** Listing of normal ranges determined for the routine hematology tests performed in the laboratory. *(Courtesy of the University of Texas M.D. Anderson Hospital, Department of Laboratory Medicine.)*

"hold," use of an intercom system, and writing messages. In addition, conversational techniques and manners should be reviewed. The following suggestions may help the phlebotomist communicate effectively and politely on the telephone.[3]

1. When answering the phone, the department's name should be stated. This saves time for both parties on the phone in case of a wrong number. In addition, some hospitals require that the employee state his or her name. To establish a cooperative relationship, he or she can offer a statement such as "May I help you?" and/or "Thank you" at the end of the conversation.

2. The tone of voice is important in conveying a message and attitude about one's work. Because the phlebotomist represents the entire clinical laboratory, it is recommended that he or she be conscious of his or her own mood when answering the telephone. For example, just because a phlebotomist has had a difficult day at work does not mean that a negative attitude should be communicated to an innocent individual at the other end of the phone line.

3. Language in a hospital setting is very specialized and words are often difficult to pronounce. To avoid problems, the communicator should use appropriate terminology for the receiving individual. The phlebotomist should use words that are concise, direct, and uncomplicated. A simple explanation or definition may clarify or prevent a misunderstanding. Spelling a term may help the receiver understand or recognize what is being said.

4. Good listening habits also function in effective communications by gaining additional information about a problem, checking word meaning, conveying a cooperative attitude, and bringing the exact message into focus. Listening techniques which may help are as follows:
   a. Restating a sentence tells the communicator that one is actually hearing the correct message.
   b. Clarifying word usage also reassures the communicator that the correct message is being transmitted.
   c. Remaining neutral in a controversy helps maintain objectivity. If one gets angry, the emotion may confuse or alter what is really being said.
   d. Reflecting on the message for a moment rather than thinking about immediate response will reinforce it. However, too much silence may indicate lack of interest.
   e. Summarizing the message back to the communicator assures that it is correct and that both parties have fully understood and are in agreement about what was transmitted.

5. Asking pertinent questions and the ability to say "I do not know," are part of effective feedback. The communicator must realize that

all individuals they speak to are not experts. The key to effective two-way communication is understanding each other and being cooperative. If it is impossible for one party to help or understand the other, then a statement such as this one will suffice, "I am sorry, but I simply cannot help you."

The importance of the role of the phlebotomist in public relations cannot be overlooked. Open communication and mutual respect should be maintained in the daily contacts between phlebotomists, other laboratory personnel, patients, nursing, housekeeping, dietary, maintenance, purchasing, and other hospital personnel, sales representatives, and nonhospital personnel.

## COMMUNICATION WITH THE COMPUTER

The computer is rapidly becoming an essential instrument in the clinical laboratory and health-care setting, and thus, the phlebotomist needs to become acquainted with automated data processing. For example, in the clinical laboratory, the functions of a laboratory computer system include: (1) entering lists of test(s) requisitions for a patient, (2) printing patients' labels, specimen collection lists and schedules, (3) updating the laboratory specimen accession records, (4) printing lists that identify what test procedures need to be performed on patients' specimens, (5) entering test results into the computer manually or through clinical laboratory instrumentation, (6) storing test results, (7) sending laboratory results to the nursing stations, and (8) sending patient charges to the accounting office.

Different types of computers are used in the laboratory and health-care setting. Some computers are large, main-frame computers that occupy usually two or more rooms and others are small microcomputers that sit on a desk top. All computers are composed of the same basic units that can transmit information, store information, and perform various types of calculations. The computer system has three main components: (1) central processing unit (CPU), (2) main memory, and (3) peripheral devices. The CPU is the heart of the computer system which performs the arithmetic operations and regulates the functions and sequence of events in the system. The main memory is the means by which the CPU stores data and programs for immediate use.

Two types of memories frequently referred to in minicomputers and microcomputers are read only memory (ROM) and read access memory (RAM). ROM is designed so that the memory is prewritten prior to being permanently placed in the computer. The memorized data are then read as needed by the computer. When the electrical power is switched off, ROM continues to store data. RAM is the memory that can be read and written by the computer as it operates. This type of memory is volatile in that the data and information are lost when the power is turned off.

Peripheral devices are devices that the computer uses for input, output, and secondary storage. Some peripherals that are used in computer systems include diskettes, card readers, magnetic tapes, printers, and video terminals sometimes referred to as the cathode ray tube (CRT).

A computer accepts input of information into its memory through messages referred to as bits and bytes. A bit (BInary digiT) is an on–off signal given in numeric language to the computer system. A numeric code of eight bits of computer language inserted into the computer is referred to as a BYTE because eight bits of information equals one byte.

The insertion of numeric codes in the computer via "bits" and "bytes" is machine language. Technology has made it possible for various computer languages to be used for communication with the computer rather than insertion of numeric codes. These languages have been developed at various times by various companies and universities to perform different types of problems. Some of the languages include: (1) FORTRAN (FORmula TRANslation)—designed to deal with scientific formulas, (2) COBOL (COmmon Business Oriented Languages)—initially devised for business applications, and (3) BASIC (Beginner's All-purpose Symbolic Instruction Code)—designed as a simple language for beginners in computer programming.

With major advances in computer technology, the phlebotomist sooner or later will become initiated to automated data processing by computerization. Thus, he or she should become thoroughly acquainted with computer terminology to provide quality health-care services through effective communication networks. Some examples of computerization in the laboratory are given later in this chapter.

## REQUISITION FORMS

The entire process of communication with which a phlebotomist becomes involved, begins the moment the laboratory is notified of a requested test. This notification is done by the laboratory requisition form. Therefore, the information or instructions on the requisition must be explicit and the design and format of the request forms to be used must be carefully considered in order to minimize handwriting, permit convenient handling, and generate inexpensive and legible copies.

Multiple-part forms, which serve both as request and report forms, represent one of the most widely used formats for a manual hospital laboratory communication system. The forms are usually of a convenient size to be easily attached to 8½ × 11 inch paper as is customarily used for patient records. Also, these forms are easy to transport, handle, sort, and store, as well as being cost-effective. For example, the forms designed for use at the University of Texas System Cancer Center, M.D. Anderson Hospital, Houston, Texas, are 3¼ inches in width by 7⅜ inch in length and are usually positioned horizontally as seen on the Hematology and Coagulation request forms in Figure 7-6. Each form is divided into sections, one side for request information and the other for results. The information on the request side (physician's name, collection time, date, clinic section, etc.) is arranged so that it always appears in the same order. This consistency allows standardization between departments and facilitates correct usage. The request information must designate time specifications, or the promptness with which the test results are needed—"stat," "routine," and so on; patient condition specifications or the circumstances at the time of specimen collection—"pre-op," "admission," as well as patient category

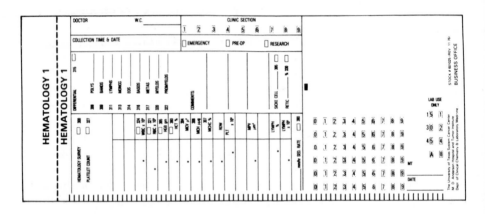

**Figure 7-6.** Multiple-part request forms which also serve as report forms. These forms are used with a computerized reporting system, but are designed to serve as temporary report forms on a "back-up" basis. *(Courtesy of the University of Texas M.D. Anderson Hospital, Department of Laboratory Medicine.)*

specifications such as "inpatient" or "outpatient." The request side also allows room for all patient identification information, whether done by means of an addressograph machine or handwritten. Each form is identified by name (Hematology 1, Coagulation, Chemistry 1, etc.) and is divided into test categories usually coinciding with the different sections of the laboratory. They are manufactured to provide clear copies (carbon paper) and easy detachment (perforated edges). Color coding can be used between request forms for ease of identification, both in the ordering of tests and in the charting of results. The name of the institution is usually included on each request form.

Certain additional specifications may be included on request slips that are to be used with a laboratory computer system or with instrumentation which generates printed results. Some request slips include a "mark-sense" top copy which is to be marked in pencil and fed through a card reader. The card reader picks up all the pencil marks and allows for the automatic entry into the computer of all requested tests for that particular patient. The patient is identified by an addressograph label containing the information routinely needed (see Patient Identification in Chapter 4) as well as by marking numbered boxes corresponding with the patient's hospital number (Fig. 7-6). Some request forms are used with a computerized reporting system, but are designed to serve also as a temporary report form on a back-up basis. Exact spacing specifications must be met when the request form is to be used as a print-out report for certain test results, as in the case of a complete blood count (CBC) as seen in Figure 7-14.

## TRANSMITTING THE TEST REQUEST TO THE LABORATORY

The request mechanism formally initiates the cyclic procedure of the patient–physician–laboratory communication network. Two systems are commonly used for this activity. Orders for test requests can be transmitted directly to the clinical laboratory from the requesting authority via an on-line interactive computer system. In many institutions, however, manual requesting systems are still in use, either utilizing mark-sense cards which are then entered into the computer, or by a totally manual request system in which the request form also serves a dual purpose as the final report.

On-line computer input of request information is the most error-free means of making requests. Because computer systems have the capability of performing automatic checks on the input, it does not accept a request for any test not in its test-information data base. Likewise, it does not accept a sample of plasma or urine for a test restricted to serum. It also allows the person entering the test request to obtain accurate and up-to-date information about specific determinations, such as revised specimen collection requirements, delivery instructions, assay techniques, normal values, and even charge fees.

In a manual system, the request forms are commonly completed at each patient unit or nursing station by a nurse or ward clerk, and delivered to the laboratory. This type of system is more subject to human error. The requisitions could be lost by the nursing service or ward clerk prior to arriving in the clinical laboratory or by the laboratory personnel after they reach the laboratory. Another common source of error comes from requests that are prepared in duplicate or not at all due to lack of communication on the nursing unit. These problems can be minimized by instituting a few organizational procedures. Providing a central location in the laboratory where all requisitions are to be delivered or scheduling laboratory personnel to make designated pick-ups of all request slips usually alleviates the problem of misplaced or lost forms. A sorting system is maintained once the requisitions reach the laboratory. The problem of whether or not a request slip has been made can be solved by including an additional copy in the request form, which can be kept on the patient unit as a record of the test requested. A blood collection log sheet at the nurses' station can also be used for this purpose. The request slips are kept with the blood collection log and compared by the phlebotomist when the blood is drawn. This system also provides the added advantage of allowing the phlebotomist to make comments on the log sheet regarding problems in obtaining the blood specimens and provides a means of communicating this to the nursing personnel.

One system that works extremely well at University of Texas M.D. Anderson Hospital and alleviates errors in test requesting involves personnel that are trained and employed by the hospital clinical laboratory but stationed at the various nursing units in a phlebotomy/liaison capacity. The formal name of the program is the Laboratory Liaison Technician (LLT) program. It was designed to maintain open and accurate communications pertaining to laboratory services with physicians, nursing service, ward clerks, patients, and family members. The LLTs are mainly responsible for the collection of all blood work requested on their assigned unit after the 7:00 AM morning draw, and for delivery of these specimens to the laboratory, as well as all other specimens. They maintain a log of all specimens collected (Fig. 7-7) and review patient charts to ensure that the laboratory tests have been accurately transcribed to the request slips. The transcription process is begun by the physician who initially requests tests to be performed on a scheduled basis or as a one-time order. Only the scheduled tests are transferred to a cardex (or Rollodex system), alleviating the necessity of the ward clerk to check each patient chart daily prior to filling out request slips. One-time laboratory orders are transcribed directly from the chart to the requisition. Any changes made by the physician regarding these initial orders are flagged on the patient's chart by a color-coded sticker notifying the unit clerk to such a change. It is easy to see how the interven-

LLT DAILY WORK SHEET

UNIT _____ DATE _____ LLT _____

TOTAL PATIENT SERVICES                                       7:00-4:00
(# OF VENIPUNCTURES)          _____ TOTAL STAT SAMPLES _____  _____

TOTAL TIMED SAMPLES _____                          3:00-11:00 _____

| ROOM # | PATIENT'S NAME | PATIENT # | TESTS TO BE DONE OR SPECIMENS DELIVERED | LOGGED BY | TIME TO BE COLLECTED | TIME COLLECTED | OBTAINED BY | SPECIMEN | COMMENT |
|--------|----------------|-----------|------------------------------------------|-----------|----------------------|----------------|-------------|----------|---------|
|        |                |           |                                          |           |                      |                |             |          |         |
|        |                |           |                                          |           |                      |                |             |          |         |
|        |                |           |                                          |           |                      |                |             |          |         |
|        |                |           |                                          |           |                      |                |             |          |         |
|        |                |           |                                          |           |                      |                |             |          |         |
|        |                |           |                                          |           |                      |                |             |          |         |
|        |                |           |                                          |           |                      |                |             |          |         |
|        |                |           |                                          |           |                      |                |             |          |         |
|        |                |           |                                          |           |                      |                |             |          |         |
|        |                |           |                                          |           |                      |                |             |          |         |
|        |                |           |                                          |           |                      |                |             |          |         |
|        |                |           |                                          |           |                      |                |             |          |         |

**Figure 7-7.** Daily log sheet documenting all specimens collected and/or delivered by the specialized phlebotomy personnel, LLTs (Laboratory Liaison Technicians). *(Courtesy of the University of Texas M.D. Anderson Hospital, Department of Laboratory Medicine.)*

tion of personnel such as an LLT could alleviate problems encountered in request transcription, request delivery, specimen collection, and so forth. Other important functions served by these specialized phlebotomists are incorporated in Figure 7-8. Specific instructions for requesting laboratory work or ordering blood products may be included in both a laboratory Bulletin of Information issued to each nursing unit and in an Administrative Services Manual issued to unit clerks. This is a good way of ensuring the proper handling of specimens and requisitions. (Refer to Fig. 7-9 for an example.)

Verbal test requests are occasionally used in cases of emergency. The request should be documented on a standardized form in the laboratory prior to the collection of the blood specimen (Fig. 7-10). After the blood has been collected, the formal laboratory request slip can be filled out and accompany the specimen to the laboratory in the routine manner.

## SPECIMEN LABELS

Clear and accurate specimen identification is essential and must begin immediately upon collection and continue through disposal of the specimen. Identification methods vary from manually copying all patient identification onto the container to utilizing prenumbered labels. Manually labeling specimens can be time consuming and usually contains errors.

---

### LLT DUTIES

1. Blood Collection -- within laboratory guidelines.

2. Deliver all Laboratory Medicine specimens to labs.

3. Deliver reports to assigned nursing units.

4. Maintain a daily log of all specimens collected.

5. Reviews patient charts as pertains to Laboratory orders.

6. Reviews ward clerks' cardex for Laboratory orders.

7. Assist I.V. Team with collection of lab specimens.

8. Advises nursing personnel on special collection techniques.

9. Serves as an information source regarding status of tests and retrieval of data from computer terminals.

10. Advises nursing staff on laboratory procedures and/or laboratory policy changes which will affect nursing.

11. Advises laboratory on laboratory needs of nursing and medical staff.

12. Works with Unit Managers in the orientation of Ward Clerks to Laboratory procedures.

13. Review nurses' cardex as pertaining to test ordered.

14. Securing print-outs of reports as they are needed.

15. Coordinating lab collections to decrease the number of venipunctures.

16. Keep floors stocked with blood collecting supplies.

17. Maintaining communications with patients and patient's family as pertaining to lab work.

---

**Figure 7-8.** Listing of specific responsibilities and duties delegated to the specialized phlebotomy personnel or the LLTs. *(Courtesy of the University of Texas M.D. Anderson Hospital, Department of Laboratory Medicine.)*

This can be avoided by using preprinted labels which are available from several sources. The Ident-a-blood* system is one request/report form that can be purchased. These contain gummed hospital labels which can be attached to specimens. Available wristband systems include those that contain gummed labels, as well as those which can imprint or electronically print patient identification information onto the specimen.

The most sophisticated, accurate, and efficient labels are those gener-

---

*Blood Identification System, Fenwal, Inc., Chicago, Illinois.

THE UNIVERSITY OF TEXAS
M. D. ANDERSON HOSPITAL AND TUMOR INSTITUTE AT HOUSTON

HOSPITAL ADMINISTRATIVE SERVICES
UNIT CLERK MANUAL


REQUESTING LABORATORY WORK

Most laboratory work is ordered on the computer readable request forms. Tests are requested by blacking out the proper box with a pencil. The name of the physician ordering the test must always be noted on the requisition form.

I.  To Order a Test on the Computer Readable Cards:

    A.  Use a #2 pencil to blackout the appropriate box. Only tests pre-printed on the request card can be ordered on each reque~ card.
    B.  Emboss each card with the appropriate patient's addressograph plate.
    C.  Pencil in the patient's hospital number in the lower right hand section of the card.

        1.  There are six rows of numbers of 0-9 on each horizontal row.
        2.  Fill in only one box per horizontal row.
        3.  Start with top row for a six digit number and work down.
        4.  Start with second row from the top for a five digit number.

    D.  Complete all information in the upper left section of the card.

        1.  Ordering Physician.
        2.  Date and time to be drawn.
        3.  Source of specimen (if requested).
        4.  Initials of the unit clerk completing and requisition.

    E.  Indicate if Pre-op or Emergency.
    F.  If you make a mistake, do not erase. Start with a new request.
    G.  Stamp in red ink: Isolation, Precaution, or Blood Precaution, (if applicable).

II.  To Order a Test not on the Computer Readable Cards:

    A.  Use a black ink pen to complete the request.
    B.  Emboss the special test requisition with the patient's addresso-graph card.
    C.  In the upper left section, indicate the order physician, and the date to be drawn.
    D.  Write in the test name and number for each test requested. Test numbers may be obtained from the Laboratory Manual on each unit.
    E.  Stamp in red ink: Isolation, Precaution, or Blood Precaution, (if applicable).

III.  Delivery of Requisitions:

    A.  Requisition for routine lab tests are picked up from the units by laboratory personnel between 1500 and 1600 and between 0000 and 0100.
    B.  Test ordered after 0100 for the same day must be hand-carried to the Laboratory Data Processing Office, Room C3.009, by the Unit Clerk or the Night Orderly.

**Figure 7-9.** Procedure for requesting laboratory tests included in the Administrative Services Manual issued to all unit clerks. *(Courtesy of the University of Texas M.D. Anderson Hospital, Department of Laboratory Medicine.)*

---

**STAT**

NURSE SIGNATURE _____

DR. REQUESTING _____

---

STAT COLLECTION REQUEST

---

LOCATION: POCU ☐     OTHER: _____

---

PATIENT:                    ROOM _____

                           PT. # _____

---

PICK UP ORDERS ON UNIT ☐

---

TESTS ORDERED:

_____

_____

_____

_____

_____

                REQUESTED  BY; _____

                ORDER  TAKEN  BY: _____

                DATE _____

                TIME ____ A.M. ____ P.M. __

---

**Figure 7-10.** Documentation form used by the laboratory in cases of verbal test results. *(Courtesy of the University of Texas M.D. Anderson Hospital, Department of Laboratory Medicine.)*

ated by a hospital computer system. Requisition slips for the morning draw can be sent to the laboratory in the afternoon of the previous day. Based on the requisition slips, the computer can generate enough labels containing all the appropriate patient identification criteria for each tube required to be drawn. The labels also contain the specific tests requested, the specimen collection tubes required for the requested tests, and unique accession numbers or sample numbers to be used for that particular collection time as shown in Figure 7-11. Transfer labels may be used to label special ali-

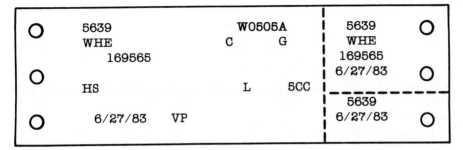

**Figure 7-11.** Computer generated labels for use by the phlebotomist during blood collection. A primary label and a "transfer" label are each printed with appropriate patient information. *(Courtesy of the University of Texas M.D. Anderson Hospital, Department of Laboratory Medicine.)*

quots, tubes, cuvettes, slides, and others. This type of system eliminates the manually written entry log used by many hospitals to record the tests requested on each patient and assigns an accession number. Additional tests ordered later in the day are entered into the computer which assigns a specific time to the tests, so they can be easily separated from the morning draw. Labels for later collection can be computer-printed or made with an addressograph. Blood drawing lists are also printed by the computer to provide a list of patients on each floor requiring blood work for the morning draw, what tests are ordered, and to identify the assigned sample number as shown in Figure 7-12. The phlebotomist initials this list after the patient's blood has been drawn and a copy is left on the floor so those attending the patient can see what tests have been collected. Any additional specimens collected later in the day are written into the log book on the floor (see Fig. 7-7). In this way, those on the floor have a complete list of the tests collected on each patient throughout the day.

Computerization of the collection process can significantly decrease errors. Without a computer, collection and specimen information must pass through several people before the sample is actually processed in the laboratory. With a computer, data are continually being checked against the computer files and each person involved can add to and receive information from it.

## SPECIMEN TRANSPORTATION AND DELIVERY

Both the communication cycle and the quality of laboratory tests results are dependent upon the time that specimens are received for processing. Phlebotomists should assure that blood and other specimens are delivered expeditiously. However, specimen transportation procedures may vary considerably between institutions.

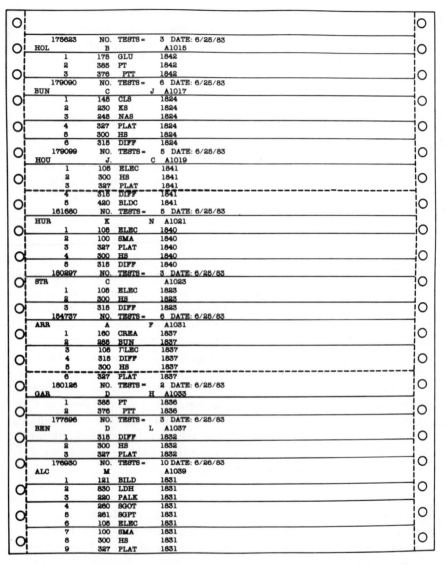

**Figure 7-12.** This is a computer-generated listing of patients on a particular unit or floor who require early morning draws. The appropriate laboratory tests are listed under each name. *(Courtesy of the University of Texas M.D. Anderson Hospital, Department of Laboratory Medicine.)*

## Hand Delivery

Many systems for specimen delivery involve hand-carried specimens and require standards for assuring promptness. The laboratory is most often the department responsible for the collection and delivery of blood specimens. The laboratory may also be responsible for the delivery of all other patient specimens as well. Phlebotomists, especially those permanently assigned to specific floors, as in the previously mentioned LLT system, can make scheduled pick-ups as well as delivery of "STAT" specimens. The specimens should be placed in an assigned area on each patient unit after being written into the log book. The patient's name, hospital number, room number, specimens delivered, time, and initials of the person transporting the specimen should be included on the log sheet as specified in Figure 7-7. Specimen transportation can be more easily monitored when all personnel involved use the appropriate documentation procedures and communicate openly with one another.

Most phlebotomists organize their blood collection trays or carts to accommodate patient specimens that need to be taken to the laboratory. A test tube rack, slide rack, plastic holder, or cup are sufficient to hold the collected specimen. Some specimens require ice for transport so it is wise to carry a small container which will not leak and fit conveniently on the tray.

## Transportation Department

Specimen delivery may also be performed by a transportation department within the hospital. When a specimen and requisition form are to be delivered to the laboratory by the transportation department, the following information is usually required: type of specimen, name and hospital identification number of the patient, date and time of specimen collection, and destination of the specimen. After obtaining this information, the escort takes the specimen to the laboratory and logs it in on a log sheet as shown in Figure 7-13. The test request slip accompanying the specimen can also be "clocked-in" at this time so that actual delivery time can always be obtained. If any complications arise with the specimen, the escort notifies the nursing unit. Occasionally, specimens, especially "STAT" or timed requests, may be collected and delivered to the laboratory by a nurse or physician. Again, the requisition should be "clocked-in."

## Pneumatic Tube System

These are used by some hospitals to transport patient records, messages, letters, bills, medications, x-rays, and laboratory results. However, reports from health-care institutions differ as to the effectiveness of using tube systems for transporting blood specimens. Some reports indicate that certain test values are affected as a result of transporting specimens in pneumatic systems. Others report that with careful evaluation and utilization of the system, it can be a time-saving and cost-effective process.[4] The Mayo Clinic reports evaluating several aspects of a pneumatic system before employing it for transporting laboratory specimens. Among these are: mechanical reliability, distance of transport, speed of carrier, control mechanisms, a soft landing mechanism, radius of loops and bends, shock absorbancy and sizes of carriers, and laboratory assessment of chemical and cellular components in transported specimens versus hand carried specimens.[4] It is gener-

| SPECIMEN DELIVERY | | | | | | | | | | |
|---|---|---|---|---|---|---|---|---|---|---|
| Patient Name | Location | Specimens | | | | | | Date | Time | Escort Name |
| | | CSF | Blood | Urine | Sputum | Other | Test Ordered | | | |
| | | | | | | | | | | |
| | | | | | | | | | | |
| | | | | | | | | | | |
| | | | | | | | | | | |
| | | | | | | | | | | |
| | | | | | | | | | | |
| | | | | | | | | | | |
| | | | | | | | | | | |
| | | | | | | | | | | |
| | | | | | | | | | | |
| | | | | | | | | | | |
| | | | | | | | | | | |
| | | | | | | | | | | |
| | | | | | | | | | | |
| | | | | | | | | | | |
| | | | | | | | | | | |
| | | | | | | | | | | |
| | | | | | | | | | | |
| | | | | | | | | | | |
| | | | | | | | | | | |

**Figure 7-13.** Log sheet used by the laboratory to document delivery of patient specimens by the institutional transport service. *(Courtesy of the University of Texas M.D. Anderson Hospital, Department of Laboratory Medicine.)*

ally recommended that blood collection tubes be placed in the pneumatic tube with shock absorbent inserts padding the sides and separated from each other to avoid spillage or breakage.

## Other Transport Equipment

Phlebotomists may also be required to order and use special transport containers. All should be evaluated for cost, protective ability, temperature control, sterilizing potential, appearance, labeling system, breakage, and leakage.

Some hospitals send specimens to reference laboratories for special analysis. When packaging or receiving one of the specimens in a special transport container, care must be taken to adhere to the following appropriate precautions:

1. Specimens such as human or animal feces, blood, body fluids, or tissue should be properly labeled and in containers that protect individuals from contamination.
2. Specimens containing viable microorganisms must be specially packaged so they can withstand leakage of contents, pressure and

temperature changes, and rough handling. It is recommended that the specimen be placed in a "primary container" surrounded by absorbant packing material. If the contents were released, they would be maintained in the "primary container." It should be labeled with pertinent information and instructions about the specimen contents. It can then be placed in a secondary container. Biohazardous and mailing labels should be affixed to the outside container.[4]

3. Specimen requisition forms or special instructions should accompany the specimen. (See also Figure 9-1.)
4. Containers holding dry ice should be labeled, e.g., "DRY ICE, FROZEN MEDICAL SPECIMEN."
5. It is recommended that, when shipping biohazardous material, the address and phone number of the Center for Disease Control, Atlanta, Georgia, be affixed to the container in the event of damage or leakage. Individuals outside the health professions may need advice on how to dispose of or clean up a biohazardous spill.
6. After receiving an intact specimen from an outside source, the container must be identified by name, number, and source. It should match the accompanying requisition and can then be processed accordingly.
7. If a leaky or broken specimen is received, it should be handled cautiously and according to safety procedures as indicated in Chapters 6 and 9.

## REPORTING MECHANISMS

### Written Reports
The laboratory report is a feedback mechanism for transmitting vital data from the laboratory to the physician requesting the information. Both the Joint Commission of Accreditation of Hospitals (JCAH) and the College of American Pathologists (CAP) state that the results should be confirmed, dated, and accompanied by permanent report copies which are kept in the laboratory as well as sent to the patient's chart. CAP also states that each report should contain adequate patient identification, be stamped to record the date and hour the procedures were completed, and be signed and initialed by the laboratory personnel performing the procedure. When computer-generated report forms are utilized, laboratory documentation on worksheets of those performing the procedures is sufficient. CAP has suggested the following qualities be included or considered when designing a report form:

1. Identification of patient, patient location, and physician
2. Date and time of specimen collection

3. Description and source of specimen when necessary
4. Compactness and ease of preparation
5. Consistency in format
6. Clear understandability
7. Logical location in patient's chart
8. Sequential order of multiple results on single specimens
9. Listing of normal ranges or normal and abnormal values
10. Assurance of accuracy of transcription of request
11. Administrative and record keeping value.[1]

Any unique institutional requirements needed for an acceptable report should be stated in the laboratory procedure manual and may include such criteria as quality control limits, absolute limits, and delta checks.[5] If these criteria cannot be met on the report form, a written policy including these requirements should be available when needed.

Results can be documented in one of the following three ways: manual recording of test results, laboratory instrument printed reports, and computer-generated reports. As previously mentioned, in most manual systems, combination test requisitioning/report forms are used. These contain multiple carbon copies as depicted in Figure 7-6. Microprocessors are in wide use today in some laboratory instruments which can generate digital outputs and printed reports as in Figure 7-14. Example of computer-generated reports are shown in Figure 7-15.

## Verbal Reports
Verbal reports, although useful for reporting "STAT" results and panic values, may become a problem in laboratories. The possibility of error is so great that at the very minimum, a laboratory should always require proper identification of the patient and the name of the person receiving the report. Written documentation of verbally issued reports is recommended and should include the following information: patient name and hospital number, person receiving the information, date, information given, and person issuing the report (Fig. 7-16.)

## Computer Reports
Various computer transmission devices can provide a rapid on-line report system, and are, in general, more reliable than verbal reports, as well as being faster than waiting for the written report. A hospital with an on-line laboratory computer system can have terminals located at each patient unit. After the tests have been completed and verified in the laboratory, the results can be immediately displayed on each patient unit. A printer can be attached to each terminal to generate a temporary hard-copy report. Another transmission method electronically transmits a hand-written

| COULTER | HEMATOLOGY | CMS # |
|---|---|---|
| # 7546613 | | 084-343 |

© 1980 COULTER ELECTRONICS, INC., HIALEAH, FLORIDA

TEST: ☐ CBC PROFILE: ☐ WBC ☐ RBC ☐ PLT ☐ PLOT

| REQ'D BY: | | DATE |
|---|---|---|
| PERFORMED BY: | | DATE |

| 0 6 / 2 6 / 8 3 | TEST NO. | 0 5 1 |
|---|---|---|

| SA | OP CODES | NORMAL VALUES |
|---|---|---|
| 8 . 0 | WBC ×10³ | M F 7.8 ± 3 |
| 3 . 4 9 | RBC ×10⁶ | M 5.4 ± 0.7 F 4.8 ± 0.6 |
| 1 0 . 8 | Hgb g/dl | M 16.0 ± 2 F 14.0 ± 2 |
| 3 2 . 4 | Hct % | M 47 ± 5 F 42 ± 5 |
| 9 2 . 6 | MCV μm³ | M 87 ± 7 F 90 ± 9 |
| 3 1 . 0 | MCH pg | M F 29 ± 2 |
| 3 3 . 4 | MCHC g/dl | M F 35 ± 2 |
| 1 6 . 8 | RDW % | M F 13 ± 1.5 |
| 2 8 5 . | PLT ×10³ | M F 130-400 |
| | | |
| 7 . 2 | MPV μm³ | M F 8.9 ± 1.5 |
| | | |
| . . . . | LYMPH % | M F 28 ± 13 |
| . . . . | LYMPH ×10³ | M F 2.0 ± 1 |

| W H I T E | Segs | | R B C | S I Z E | Norm |
|---|---|---|---|---|---|
| | Bands | | | | Micro |
| | Eos | | | | Macro |
| | Basos | | M O R P H. | C O L O R | Norm |
| E | Lymphs | | | | Hypo |
| C E L L S | Monos | | | | Poly |
| | Atyp. Lym. | | | S H A P E | Norm |
| | Imm. Gran. | | | | Poik |
| | Blasts | | PLATELETS | Inc. | Nml. | Dec. |
| % | Other | | Appear | | | |
| NRBC/100 WBC | | | Plt. Est. × 10³ | | | |
| WBC Est. × 10³ | | | TEST NO. | | | |
| Review Code | | | | | | |

COMMENTS:

LABORATORY COPY

**Figure 7-14.** Hematology report form with results printed by a laboratory instrument. This type of form may be used both as a request form and as a final report form. *(Adapted from Coulter Electronics, Inc. Hialeah, Florida, with permission.)*

LABORATORY MEDICINE, M. D. ANDERSON HOSPITAL AND TUMOR INSTITUTE

| TEST NAME | RESULT | UNITS | TEST NAME | RESULT | UNITS |
|---|---|---|---|---|---|
| •HEMATOLOGY SURVEY | | | MYELOCYTE | 3 | % |
| WBC COUNT | 0.6 | K/UL | •PLATELET COUNT | 26. | K/UL |
| RED BLOOD CELL COUNT | 2.37 | M/UL | ABS GRAN (K) | 0.20 | |
| HEMOGLOBIN | 7.3 | G/DL | ABS LEUK (K) | 0.00 | |
| HEMATOCRIT | 20.5 | % | | | |
| MCV | 86 | FL | | | |
| MCH | 31.0 | PG | | | |
| MCHC | 35.8 | G/DL | | | |
| •DIFFERENTIAL COUNT | 33 | | | | |
| PLAT DECRES | | | | | |
| POLYS | 33 | % | | | |
| LYMPH | 60 | % | | | |
| MONO | 3 | % | | | |

REPORTED:1943 7/3/83 TEC: 59:218: 59: 0: 3758

FRA W. 180035 M0310 SPEC. COLLECTED: 702 7/3/83

TEST CHARGES: $34.00 HEMATOLOGY

**Figure 7-15.** Computer-generated report form with hematology test results. *(Courtesy of the University of Texas M.D. Anderson Hospital, Department of Laboratory Medicine.)*

**CULTURE RESULTS—PHONE REQUEST**

**NECESSARY INFORMATION

PATIENT NAME ____________________

PATIENT NUMBER ____________________

PERSON REQUESTING INFORMATION ____________________

| DATE | SOURCE | CULTURE # | INFORMATION GIVEN |
|---|---|---|---|

DATE OF INQUIRY AND TECHNOLOGIST ____________________

**Figure 7-16.** Form used by the microbiology laboratory for documentation of culture reports issued verbally. *(Courtesy of the University of Texas M.D. Anderson Hospital, Department of Laboratory Medicine.)*

report which is generated in a similar form at the receiving end. A third transmission device transmits facsimile results, similar to a Xerox copy of the report, to an output device. All of these methods can provide a written report which is usually accurate, dependable, and consistent.

## DISTRIBUTION OF RESULTS

The final communication involved in the patient–physician–laboratory cycle is the distribution of test results. Those who receive the laboratory data include nursing and medical record personnel (chart attachment), the hospital business office (patient billing), and the laboratory (department record).

In order to provide a chronological type of reporting system in the patient's chart, the laboratory reports are usually shingled one upon another. Color coding by the laboratory originating the results aids in coordinating them on a carrier page. The laboratory may also key chronological reports by having a master card prepared in the laboratory for each patient, beginning with the admitting laboratory results. The results of each day are added to the card which can be photocopied and sent to the physician. This also allows the laboratory without a computer system to perform delta checks on the results before releasing them.[5] A hospital computer system can easily provide daily printed reports and cumulative reports for the patient's chart. All reports should be printed and delivered at times convenient for mounting on the chart and should also be suited to the schedule of the medical staff. Some hospitals send a second set of results directly to the physician in case errors or delays in chart attachments occur. This helps to ensure that the data are available to the physicians before making patient rounds.

The business office of the hospital also receives laboratory results. They must be notified of all laboratory charges, according to data requested, for patient billing. It is advantageous to send reports promptly so the patient can avoid late charges, which generate patient complaints.

Laboratory copies of test results must be maintained in storage because data from previous days, months, or years are often requested. A copy of the combined request/report form can be easily stored and used for information retrieval. In a manual reporting system, log books are often kept in the laboratory and usually serve as duplicate recording of patient results. They can be beneficial in permitting a more rapid retrieval of a patient's previous results and aid in providing a delta check procedure. Computer systems can store easily retrievable information for long periods of time, require no paperwork from laboratory personnel, and can be programmed to automatically display and flag delta checks.

## STUDY QUESTIONS

1. Identify 6 ways to enhance intralaboratory communications.
2. Describe guidelines for designing a requisition/report form.
3. Name 3 ways commonly used to transport specimens.
4. Name areas or departments that usually receive laboratory reports.
5. What is the mechanism that formally initiates the patient–physician–laboratory communication cycle?
6. What is the most error-free method of test requisitioning and why?
7. What is the most important guideline to be followed when obtaining a blood specimen from a patient?

## REFERENCES

1. College of American Pathologists: Standards for Accreditation of Medical Laboratories. Skokie, Ill., College of American Pathologists, 1974.
2. Becan-McBride K (ed): Textbook of Clinical Laboratory Supervision. New York, Appleton-Century-Crofts, 1982.
3. Martin BG, Viskochil KR, Amos PA (eds): Clinical Laboratory Management, A Guide for Clinical Laboratory Scientists. Boston, Little, Brown, 1982.
4. Slockbauer JM, Blumenfeld TA: Collection and Handling of Laboratory Specimens, A Practical Guide. St. Louis, J.B. Lippincott, 1983.
5. Henry J (ed): Clinical Diagnosis and Management by Laboratory Methods. Philadelphia, Saunders, 1979.
6. Inhorn S (ed): Quality Assurance Practice for Health Laboratories. Washington, D.C., American Public Health Association, 1978.
7. JCAH Accreditation Manual for Hospitals: Chicago, Joint Commission on Accreditation of Hospitals, 1976.
8. Newell J: Laboratory Management. Boston, Little, Brown, 1972.
9. Shuffstall R, Hemmaplardh B: The Hospital Laboratory. St. Louis, Mosby, 1979.
10. University of Texas System Cancer Center, M.D. Anderson Hospital and Tumor Institute, Hospital Administrative Services Unit Clerk Manual, 1982.
11. University of Texas System Cancer Center, M.D. Anderson Hospital and Tumor Institute, Laboratory Bulletin of Information, 1982.
12. University of Texas System Cancer Center, M.D. Anderson Hospital and Tumor Institute, Laboratory Liaison Technician Manual, 1979.

# CHAPTER 8

# Interpersonal Skills and Professionalism

## Annot F. Littlepage

## PATIENT RELATIONS

As a vital member of the clinical laboratory team, the phlebotomist provides the link between the patient and the analytic area. The quality of the blood specimens determines the quality of the diagnostic test results. The ease of collection of these specimens depends upon the skills and abilities of the phlebotomist to perform the collection techniques and to interact successfully with the patient.

### Bedside Manner

The climate established by the phlebotomist upon entering a patient's room begins before he or she leaves the laboratory area. The feeling of confidence that comes from the knowledge that the collection tray is clean and completely stocked is the first step in a good bedside manner. A pleasant face, neat appearance, and professional manner set the stage for a positive encounter when dealing with patients. The first 30 seconds after the phlebotomist enters the patient's room determines how that patient perceives the clinical laboratory and· in some cases, the quality of patient care offered by that hospital. Most patients admit that the procedure they dread most is being "stuck" for blood collection.

As discussed in previous chapters, the phlebotomist should introduce him or herself as Mr.————/Ms.———— and then state that he or she is part of the hospital or laboratory staff. The patient should be informed that the specimen is being collected for a test ordered by the physician. This statement should be stressed. Also a statement that this is routine hospital protocol often reassures the patient. A lengthy discussion of why a certain test was ordered or what tests were ordered is not appropriate. These questions should be referred to the patient's physician.

During all steps of the venipuncture, the phlebotomist should remain calm and professional. Before leaving the patient, he or she should make sure the patient is alright and thank him or her for cooperating.

## Patient Interview

Hospitals and laboratories differ slightly in their guidelines for patient interviews. All agree that proper patient identification is essential. Ask the patient "What is your name?" not "Are you Ms. Smith?" A patient will often agree with anything he or she is asked. Some institutions insist that the phlebotomist ask for the patient's complete address, while others require the mention of the hometown or street to reinforce and confirm identity. Some prefer that patients spell an unusual last name. This portion of the specimen collection procedure assures that the remainder of the diagnostic testing protocol provides information on the correct person.

It is important for the phlebotomist to remember that nonverbal cues or body language plays an important part in communication in terms of what the patient perceives and how he or she responds. Nonverbal cues are particularly important in dealing with children. They may not understand the words but they can sense how adults feel about them through tone of voice and movements. A child should not be told "this won't hurt." When the procedure does hurt, the child will not believe anything else said. There is a high probability that he or she will react negatively to the next person who attempts to collect a blood sample.

A knowledge of the stages of human development[1] as shown in Table 8-1 should enable the phlebotomist to anticipate the reactions and fears expressed in childhood behavior patterns.

Anything said to parents or children should be carefully considered before speaking. It is helpful if the phlebotomist remains calm, friendly, and professional throughout the procedure because both adults and children may be apprehensive about what has happened to them. They have been removed from what is familiar, they have not been feeling well, and they do not understand why different things are done.

If the phlebotomist is assisting in the collection of blood donors, there are some essential questions that must be asked during the private prospective donor interview:

1. How long has it been since he or she has eaten? (A donor should have eaten and not been fasting for a lengthy period. If a donor has not eaten, it is recommended that he or she eat something light or a snack prior to collection.)

**TABLE 8-1. HUMAN DEVELOPMENT—MODEL[a]**

| Stage-Age | Fears/Concerns | Proper Parent Behavior |
|---|---|---|
| Newborn (0–12 months) | Totally dependent on parents/adults<br>Trust that adults respond to basic needs | Parent should hold infant as an aid to collector and to comfort child |
| Infants and toddlers (12–24 months) | Little fear of danger<br>Fear of separation from mother<br>Limited language and understanding | Parent should stay in background until blood is drawn unless asked to help |
| Pre-school (3–6 years) | Greater body awareness<br>Play years<br>Puppets = "play"<br>Explain actions in language child can understand | Parent should stay in background until blood is drawn unless asked to participate |
| School age (preadolescent) (6–12 years) | Fears loss of self-control<br>Less dependent on parent – autonomy<br>Child may be willing to participate | Child may ask parent to leave room |
| Teenager (12–18 years) | Actively involved in anything concerning the body<br>Embarrassed to show fear<br>May act hostile to mask fear | May not want to have parent present |
| Special problems Mentally retarded | Need unhurried gentle approach | Have parent/guardian stay with child. |

[a]Stages 1 – 5 are adapted from Erickson E H: Childhood and Society, 2nd ed, Norton, New York, 1963.

2. Has the donor taken any aspirin in the last 72 hours?
3. Does the donor have a cold or fever?
4. What are his or her weight, height, age?
5. Has the donor had any of the following diseases?
   a. malaria
   b. hepatitis
   c. herpes
   d. tuberculosis
   e. syphilis
5. Is he or she in any of the currently identified high risk groups of AIDS or Acquired Immune Deficiency Syndrome? These high risk groups are:
   a. patients with hemophilia;
   b. Haitian entrants to the United States;
   c. those with symptoms and signs suggestive of AIDS (rare or unusual infections such as *Pneumocystis pneumonia* or a rare skin cancer, Kaposi's sarcoma);
   d. sexual partners of AIDS patients;
   e. sexually active homosexual or bisexual men with multiple partners;
   f. sexual partner of individual at increased risk of AIDS.

Also, does he/she have any of the following?

g. unexplained weight loss of over 10 lb

h. unexplained fever

i. night sweats

j. swollen or enlarged lymph nodes.

If the answer is "yes," he or she should be asked to refrain from donating blood.

The prospective donor must have his or her blood pressure, hemoglobin or hematocrit, and temperature checked.[2]

## Patient Teaching

For some laboratory procedures to be successful, the patient must participate and cooperate. The phlebotomist must be willing and able to provide sufficient understandable instruction to the patient for protocols to be accomplished. In some clinical situations, patients with diabetes need to be instructed on the use of mechanical aids to perform fingersticks on themselves at home to check blood sugar levels.

Nursing staff or unit personnel may have instructed the inpatient that he or she will be fasting or have nothing by mouth until after the early morning blood collections. The phlebotomist should listen to patient's comments about "not having breakfast yet" or "they won't feed me." Even a question or comment about food may inspire a response to confirm that the patient was truly fasting. Even more critical are the timed tests such as the glucose tolerance test. In this test, patient understanding is essential. The patient should be informed of the following:

1. A fasting blood specimen is drawn and urine collected.
2. The fasting period is followed by a measured intake of food or a measured glucose drink.
3. After a 30-minute interval, blood is drawn and a urine specimen collected.
4. The nursing staff is advised that the time has started. Blood and urine specimens are collected at hourly intervals for 2, 3, 4, or 5 hours.

    NOTE: For the procedure to yield valid and reliable results the patient must: (a) stay fasting, (b) be in his or her room at the specified time, and (c) drink enough water to provide the timed urine specimens.

If the patient is a child, the parents or guardian must receive and understand the instructions. If the patient begins to feel ill or faint, the nursing personnel or phlebotomy supervisor should be notified. If the patient is an outpatient, the phlebotomist and other laboratory personnel must monitor the condition of the patient. A bed and bathroom must be convenient to the collection area to provide for the comfort and safety of the patient.

Another timed specimen often used in laboratory medicine is the 24-hour urine specimen. For the specimen to fit into most laboratory schedules, it is advisable to have the patient void at 7:00 AM and discard the urine. The next urine and all urine voided for 24 hours is saved in the container provided. The patient should be cautioned that to have good results *ALL* the urine must be saved or the procedure will have to be started over.

For urine cultures, the patient must be instructed in proper specimen collection techniques to insure valid results from microbiology. Occasionally, clinic patients require instruction in collection of stool specimens for culture, examination for ova and parasites, or occult blood. Also, the Scotch tape method for diagnosis of pinworms should be available in the procedure manual if needed for outpatient teaching. Although infrequent, the need to instruct the outpatient about the collection of a 24-hour stool specimen for fecal fat may be necessary.

With the advances in the area of therapeutic drug monitoring, the physician must know not only the time and date of collection but whether the blood was collected before or after medication was given. The length of time is a factor with some drugs. The future dictates coordinated drug delivery and blood collection designed with computer assistance. This type of program necessitates a readily available blood collection team or a couple of designated drug monitoring phlebotomists.

Communication of information is essential for teaching patients and for laboratory testing. However, there are barriers to understanding. For understanding and communication to take place, the entire communication loop (Fig. 8-1) must be completed.

The message must leave the sender and reach the receiver; then the receiver must provide feedback to the sender. Without feedback, the sender has no way of knowing whether or not the filters blocked the meaning of the message. Some of the most frequently encountered filters to verbal communication are

1. language,
2. handicaps such as deafness,
3. cultural differences,
4. English as a second language,
5. emotions—anger, fear, distrust,
6. age, and
7. time—not enough to insure understanding.

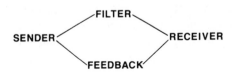

Figure 8-1. Communication loop.

*Language Barriers.* Many members of the health-care team use jargon or medical terminology to hide what they are saying from the patient. Also the meaning of words varies with the context and the age of the speaker. To promote understanding, a vocabulary that is easily understood should be used with a patient whenever possible.

*Handicaps.* The more complex the directions are, the greater the need to communicate. Thus, the phlebotomist should be more sensitive to patients who are deaf. A question like "How will you do this?" or "When will you begin to start this task?" gives better clues that the patient has heard and understood than "Do you understand?"

*Cultural Differences.* In some areas of the country the wide variety of cultures represented on the hospital staff and in the patient populations add more filters to understanding between people. To some patients, if eye contact is not established there is no truth in what is said. The phlebotomist should sense the situation and respond to the patient's needs.

*English as a Second Language.* Often patients understand from nonverbal cues, but the blood drawer must know how to locate an interpreter, if available, when the patient does not speak or comprehend English. If a large segment of the patient population speaks another language, the hospital, the laboratory staff development or continuing education program should provide basic usage of that language. In the Southwest it is important to develop some skill in the Spanish language. For basic requests in Spanish, French, and Vietnamese refer to Appendix I. It is recommended that one practices the phrases with someone who can speak the language before attempting to communicate with a patient. Mispronounced words may lead to more confusion.

*Emotions as Barriers.* Anger, fear, and distrust are all barriers to communication. If a patient is angry and refuses to have blood drawn, more time must be spent with the patient. The nurse, physician, or supervisor may be needed to try and persuade the patient to comply. The blood drawer needs to realize that the patient is often being stubborn because of emotions generated by other events. He or she may be angry because he or she cannot have morning coffee or breakfast or was awakened from a sound sleep at a very early hour. The anger is then vented on the first person that comes into the room. The phlebotomist must learn not to be upset. He or she must walk away and treat the next patient with concern and consideration. A calm, confident, and professional manner often is the best method to interact with an emotionally upset patient. A smile can set the stage for open lines of communication. Each patient is the most important person in the world at that moment in time.

*Age.* The vocabulary of a teenager is different from that of someone 70 to 80 years old. The phlebotomist must clarify the word usage for each age.

## PATIENT CARE AND MANAGEMENT

Having enough trained staff to collect the early morning draws in a hospital within a reasonable time frame is the first step in good patient care and management for the phlebotomy team. In an outpatient or clinic area, coordinated scheduling helps decrease stress levels and length of waiting time. To prepare schedules, the supervisor needs to develop data bases to include:

1. Average time for nursery stick including gowning, handwashing before entering nursery, and handwashing between infants
2. Average time for adult microcollection
3. Average time for pediatric microcollection
4. Average time of routine venipuncture
5. If the hospital or clinic is large, what is the travel time from the laboratory or blood drawing area to the patient unit, and back to receiving/processing?
6. What is the average load level on each route at any time of day?
7. When is there most activity from the emergency room?
8. To improve cooperation and scheduling, the medical staff and phlebotomy or laboratory supervisor must agree on specific items.
   a. How long before and how long after 4:00 PM can a glucose scheduled for 4:00 PM be drawn?
   b. Does the analytic area need all specimens (i.e., blood chemistry profiles) by a specific time to optimize utilization of automated equipment or available laboratory staff?
   c. What is an acceptable turnaround time for test results?
   d. Is the acceptable turnaround time possible?
   e. When are most routine blood specimens drawn?
      (See Figure 8-2.)

There should be agreements between patient units or clinical areas that a patient involved in a timed procedure should be readily available to have the specimen collected at the proper time and not be transported to radiology or physical therapy. Another facet of patient care is time management on the part of the individual phlebotomist. After cleaning the collection tray, supplies should be reviewed so that all the tubes and supplies

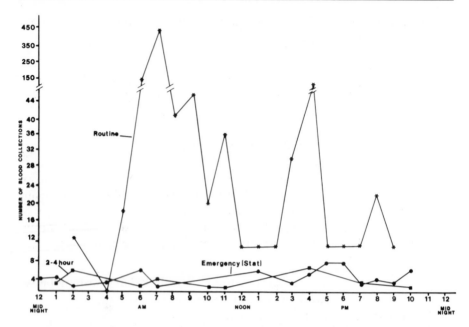

**Figure 8-2.** The graph depicts results of a study on the number of inpatient adult blood specimens collected over a one-month period on an average sized hospital floor. It shows the number and types of specimens drawn at various times of the day.

routinely needed are stocked on the tray. In an outpatient area, the cabinet or chair should be checked and stocked for the day.

To review, the basis for good patient care management includes the following:

1. Planning—supplies, routes, and staffing.
2. Availability of patient at appropriate time.
3. Knowledge of procedure and technique.
4. Confident and caring attitude when dealing with patients, health-care team members, families, and visitors.

## STAT Blood Collection

For patients in the surgical suite, recovery room, or emergency room, the phlebotomist should realize that the patients in these locations usually have the need for emergency or STAT blood collection. Patients that are in the hospital or come in for chemotherapy often have veins that have been damaged or must be avoided and used only for treatment. Each patient must be considered in terms of their individual needs not as the "burn case down the hall" or "the broken leg on 3C." As long as the phlebotomist is willing to provide care in a professional manner and respond to each patient as an individual, the quality of care will improve.

## PREPARATION FOR LABORATORY TESTING

The admitting office or the physician's office is usually the first component in preparing the patient for laboratory testing. Preadmission counseling should include background information of laboratory tests usually required during a hospital stay. For the outpatient, instruction may have been given by nursing or laboratory staff or the physician. The phlebotomist should find out what the patient already knows and build a positive atmosphere that reinforces the essential background preparation for clinical laboratory testing.

The most important information received from the patient is his or her identity. The proper identification of the blood specimen is of primary concern to the phlebotomist.

## FAMILY AND VISITORS

There are times in a busy hospital or laboratory day when families and visitors are much more difficult to deal with than patients. Often families and visitors make requests or demands that are not part of the accepted behavior for a phlebotomist.

Patients should not be given water or food without the physician's permission. Usually, it is better to inform the nurse of the patient's request. Visitors and family can be asked to step into the hall while the blood specimen is being drawn. If the phlebotomist feels that assistance is required, a family member may be asked to help.

Priests and chaplains have the right to visit privately with patients. Unless the blood specimen is timed, it is best to return to that patient after completing the other draws in the unit or area. The physician may also wish to confer privately with the patient. The same procedure as with a priest or chaplain should be followed. If the procedure is timed or "STAT," the phlebotomist may ask permission to collect the specimen.

Families and visitors of patients are not welcome in the clinical laboratory areas except by prior arrangement. Their safety and the confidentiality of patient records must be considered.

## PATIENT RIGHTS

All members of the clinical laboratory team must recognize that their first responsibility is to the patient's health, safety, and personal dignity. As given on page 194, many hospitals and other health-care facilities have incorporated "A Patients' Bill of Rights" as developed by the American Hospital Association into policy manuals. Each paragraph will be examined as it relates to the role of the phlebotomist.

## A PATIENT'S BILL OF RIGHTS*

Approved by the House of Delegates of the American Hospital Association February 6, 1973. The American Hospital Association presents a Patient's Bill of Rights with the expectation that observance of these rights will contribute to more effective patient care and greater satisfaction for the patient, his/her physician, and the hospital organization. Further, the Association presents these rights in the expectation that they will be supported by the hospital on behalf of its patients, as an integral part of the healing process. It is recognized that a personal relationship between the physician and the patient is essential for the provision of proper medical care. The traditional physician–patient relationship takes on a new dimension when care is rendered within an organizational structure. Legal precedent has established that the institution itself also has a responsibility to the patient. It is in recognition of these factors that these rights are affirmed.[3]

1. The patient has the right to considerate and respectful care.
2. The patient has the right to obtain from his/her physician complete current information concerning his/her diagnosis, treatment, and prognosis in terms the patient can be reasonably expected to understand. When it is not medically advisable to give such information to the patient, the information should be made available to an appropriate person in his/her behalf. He has the right to know by name, the physician responsible for coordinating his/her care.
3. The patient has the right to receive from his/her physician information necessary to give informed consent prior to the start of any procedure and/or treatment. Except in emergencies, such information for informed consent should include but not necessarily be limited to the specific procedure and/or treatment, the medically significant risks involved, and the probable duration of incapacitation. Where medically significant alternatives for care or treatment exist, or when the patient requests information concerning medical alternatives, the patient has the right to such information. The patient also has the right to know the name of the person responsible for the procedures and/or treatment.
4. The patient has the right to refuse treatment to the extent permitted by law, and to be informed of the medical consequences of his/her action.
5. The patient has the right to every consideration of his/her privacy concerning his/her own medical care program. Case discussion, consultation, examination, and treatment are confidential and should be conducted discreetly. Those not directly involved in his/her care must have the permission of the patient to be present.
6. The patient has the right to expect that all communications and records pertaining to his/her care should be treated as confidential.
7. The patient has the right to expect that within its capacity a hospital must make reasonable response to the request of a patient for services. The hospital must provide evaluation, service, and/or referral as indicated by the urgency of the case. When medically permissible a patient may be transferred to another facility only after he/she has received complete information and explanation concerning the needs for and alternatives to such a transfer. The institution to which the patient is to be transferred must first have accepted the patient for transfer.
8. The patient has the right to obtain information as to any relationship of his/her hospital to other health care and educational institutions insofar as his/her care is concerned. The patient has the right to obtain information as to the existence of any professional relationships among individuals, by name, who are treating him.
9. The patient has the right to be advised if the hospital proposes to engage in or perform human experimentation affecting his/her care or treatment. The patient has the right to refuse to participate in such research projects.
10. The patient has the right to expect reasonable continuity of care. He/she has the right to know in advance what appointment times and physicians are available and where. The

patient has the right to expect that the hospital will provide a mechanism whereby he/she is informed by his/her physician or a delegate of the physician of the patient's continuing health care requirements following discharge.

11. The patient has the right to examine and receive an explanation of his/her bill regardless of source of payment.
12. The patient has the right to know what hospital rules and regulations apply to his/her conduct as a patient.

*(Reprinted with permission of The American Hospital Association, copyright 1975, with permission.)*

## Review of Patient's Bill of Rights:

1. The patient may be rude, ill-tempered, and uncooperative. However, it is important for hospital personnel to deliver the best quality of care they are capable of giving, being careful to show consideration and concern for each patient.

2. Laboratory personnel are not to give misdirected or inappropriate information about laboratory tests, test results, or test procedures. This can generally be handled correctly by saying to the patient "the doctor ordered blood to be drawn for testing." This is routinely performed on admission or as a part of general care. The remainder of the questions should be directed to the physician on the case. It is the physician's decision as to how much should be told to the patient in his or her care.

3. There are basically two rights incorporated in this statement. First, as a portion of the principle of informed consent, the phlebotomist should briefly explain to the patient the procedures used to collect the blood sample. The patient also has the right to know that the blood drawing team member is part of the hospital staff and who he or she is. It is important for the phlebotomist to stress that the physician has ordered the tests. The patient also has the right to know if someone involved in their care is a student.

4. If a patient refuses to have a blood specimen drawn, it is the phlebotomist's responsibility to remind the patient that his or her physician has ordered the clinical laboratory tests performed as part of the medical care. If the patient still refuses, the phlebotomist should inform the nursing staff and, if possible, the physician. The phlebotomist should avoid any emotional confrontation or conflict with the patient.

5. Requests for certain laboratory tests and results on clinical laboratory tests are part of the patient's treatment and are confidential. This rule of confidentiality extends to other members of the clinical laboratory staff when in a public place, such as a hospital elevator or cafeteria. Some family member or friend may overhear. Also, patients, especially teenagers, have strong feelings about showing fear. Their need for privacy should be respected. If

the patient's physician is in the room and discussing treatment or disease condition, the phlebotomist should excuse him or herself and come back later unless the physician specifically requests that the blood specimen be drawn. If the phlebotomist has a "STAT" request, he or she should quietly ask the physician if he or she wishes it drawn now or wants him or her to return.

6. Clinical laboratory requisition slips contain demographic data that should not be exposed to the public even before analytic results are recorded. It is the responsibility of the hospital to provide security for data in electronic information storage and retrieval systems and make the information available only to those that have specific need. Any discussion of tests or test results on a specific patient are not appropriate in a public place. If the patient is a rational, responsible adult, then information given by his or her doctor may be shared with family and visitors by the patient or during a conference with the physician. Sometimes a very talkative patient may wish to share information of a personal and sensitive nature with the phlebotomist. It is appropriate to politely stop the patient from disclosure and continue with the collection procedure.

7. Occasionally, a patient assumes that any staff member that walks into his or her room is a nurse or nursing assistant. The patient may request a drink or help in moving. The phlebotomist should tell the patient to call a member of the nursing staff to handle the request. The phlebotomist should not give food, water, or cigarettes to a patient as these items might be counterindicated because of the patient's condition.

8. This is usually applied to one physician requesting that another physician come in as a consultant with the first physician receiving some consideration. Also, the laws and statutes require that one physician not pay another physician to become part of a case. Others feel that this applies to students. The patient has the right to know if the phlebotomist is a student. He or she has the right to refuse to be involved with students. It is important for the supervisor to reassure the patient of the student's competency to perform the procedure. In a teaching hospital or laboratory, the patient implies permission for student involvement upon admission. However, every effort should be made to have student–patient interactions as positive as possible.[4]

9. a. A patient may feel without reason that he or she may be part of experimentation. However, in most medical teaching facilities there is a Committee for the Protection of Human Subjects that reviews any experimentation that involves human subjects in any way. On some campuses there are advertisements in the campus paper for paid subjects for research. Generally they are asked to have blood drawn to help establish the normal values

range for healthy people. This may vary with the project. This also holds for behavioral research and involves the decision and legal implication of deciding who to put in the group that does not participate when the gain from participating is permanent. Many research projects in medicine use numbers in large groups with no names and thus avoid having each patient in a large group provide signed consent.

b. A patient must have the opportunity to weigh the risk factors and inconvenience against what may be learned from his or her voluntary participation.

10. Any treatment or laboratory testing ordered to aid in diagnosis or therapy will be performed in a timely manner provided the patient is willing.

11. The patient has a right to review his or her hospital bill.

12. The phlebotomist must sometimes remind a patient that special rules about test procedures are a part of hospital or diagnostic protocol and must be adhered to for successful test results.

## RESPONSIBILITIES

### Accountability

In one sense of the word, accountability is to audit and account for the money spent on people and supplies. Financial advisors or budget office personnel may insist on knowing that equipment and personnel were used and scheduled efficiently, regardless of the institutional setting.

The analytic term for accountability is quality control or the maintenance of analytic accuracy, reproducibility, and reliability. Quality control can provide data for regular critical evaluation of laboratory performance. Objective data can be calculated and classified then used for daily, monthly, or annual review.

Personal accountability, however, cannot be calculated in a mathematical equation. Each individual phlebotomist has a personal responsibility for providing quality assurance. For example, the phlebotomist is responsible for poor technique if a large number of separate specimens are hemolyzed on delivery to the laboratory. This is wasteful in the financial sense and not good patient care because of the need to redraw. Generally, the phlebotomist is not asked to account for his or her actions unless an incident report is written or a patient or other health-care team member complains. Various time logs on patient units and in the outpatient area provide documentation of performance. The validity of these is based on being conscientious and honest. Personal integrity or "doing what's right when no one is looking" (i.e., washing hands between patients, observing precautions to gown and scrub in isolation, and collecting timed tests at the proper time) are reflections on a phlebotomist's personal accountability or individual responsibility for actions. In some situations, the phlebotomist may be held legally accountable or answerable for his or her actions. If a patient sues the hospital or clinical laboratory, staff members questioned on procedure will be part of a deposition. Each member of the health-care team should have a personal commitment to fulfill the obligations imposed by the health-care system.

## Motivation and Attitude

With the growth of the industrial work place, the basic ideas about work and workers have changed. A major change in America was the movement of workers away from farms, as self-employed individuals, to factories, as cogs in the enormous mechanized system. With this change, there were other changes in the assumptions about why people are productive in a work setting. To reconstruct some of the foundations and examine current theories, a few of the recognized mile posts in human behavior follow.

*Sigmund Freud.* Dr. Freud began his studies in human behavior by investigating hysteria from a psychologic aspect. Freud published works on neurology with emphasis on cerebral paralyses of children. Hypnotism was used to treat hysteria by recall of hidden and important circumstances in patients' lives. Freud then began to use a "free association" method instead of hypnotism. His published discoveries were as follows.

1. There is an unconscious mind.
2. The unconscious has an influence on the conscious.
3. The mind is in layers.
4. The existence of infantile sexuality is important.

These ideas were met with some strong opposition, and some have been displaced as behavioral scientists learn more about human psychology, actions, and interactions.

Probably the most persistent contribution he made was the theory of the "unconscious mind." Most phlebotomists have had situations in which they felt unpleasant or uncomfortable in one area of the hospital or laboratory for no apparent reason. However, on recall the phlebotomist may remember that a patient on that unit or in that laboratory area was the cause of a traumatic personal experience.

*Hawthorne Experiment.* In the late 1920s, experiments were conducted to examine the behavior of workers in an industrial setting. These experiments were at the Hawthorne plant of the Western Electric Company. The findings were reported by Roethlisberger in his book *Management and Morale* (1941). These experiments were originally designed to study the relationship between illumination and productivity of workers. The results obtained were not those expected. A test group was subjected to various levels of lighting in the work area while the control group work area received constant illumination consistent with their normal work setting. Production increased in both groups with the same degree of increase for control and test groups, even when there were dramatic changes in lighting. There was no reduction in production until the experimental group level of lowered illumination reached "moonlight."

It appeared that illumination of the work area had no effect on productivity. However, the experimenters were not willing to accept this conclusion. Other experiments were designed and conducted over a 5-year period, and data were collected and analyzed. After years of additional study there were no results. However, after looking for further answers directly from employees over a long period of time, the tool of "interviewing" was developed. Through extensive interviewing they found:

1. Sentiments (loyalty, integrity, solidarity, etc.) and feelings influence behavior.
2. Sentiments are difficult to study because people can and often mask or disguise them.
3. The total situation of a person is a manifestation of the sentiments and personal history of that person at that one particular time.

The basic conclusion was that "the worker is a social animal," and personal sentiments can greatly affect behavior on the job. Supervisors should be sensitive to emotions and loyalties different from their own.

*Abraham H. Maslow.* In 1943, A.H. Maslow dramatically changed the theories and approaches to understanding human motivation by publishing his views. He stated[6]:

1. There are at least five sets of goals, which we call basic needs. They are briefly physiological, safety, love, esteem and self actualization. In addition, we are motivated by the desire to achieve or maintain the various conditions upon which these basic satisfactions rest and by certain more intellectual desires.
2. These basic goals are related to each other, being arranged in a hierarchy of prepotency. This means that the most prepotent will monopolize consciousness and will tend of itself to organize the recruitment of the various capacities of the organism. The less prepotent needs are minimized, even forgotten or denied.

The basic model for the hierarchy of needs that he defined can be illustrated graphically (Fig. 8-3).

Maslow suggested that when one "need" was fairly well-satisfied, it ceases becoming a motivator. At that time the next or higher need begins to dominate the center of motivation. The lines separating the various needs should be dim or blurred as there are overlaps in each area.

## Hierarchy of Human Needs

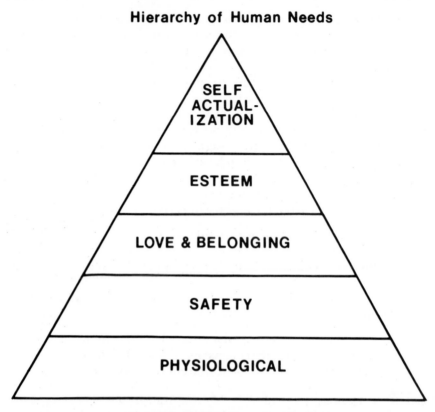

**Figure 8-3.** Maslow's Hierarchy of Needs.

*Physiologic Needs.* Physiologic needs trigger the body's automatic efforts to maintain internal body balance or equilibrium. In the clinical laboratory, this may be expressed in the blood acid—base balance, carbon dioxide content, glucose content, and oxygen content, to name only a few. A person who is lacking food, social contacts, security, and esteem would satisfy the hunger need first. The needs for air, food, and water are survival needs. These critical needs are met first and felt most strongly. In the hospital or laboratory setting, this helps to explain the behavior of the difficult patient who has been fasting or is just hungry. A man on the brink of starvation will dream of food, think of food, and work frantically to acquire food. It is almost impossible to teach or communicate with a hungry child.

*Safety Needs.* Safety needs are those which emerge as the center for action and thought after the physiologic needs have been satisfied. Because human beings have so long ignored the consequences of air, water, and general environmental pollution, federal agencies have mushroomed in response to growing fears about human safety in relation to the environment.

In general, threats by extremes of temperature, criminal violence, or vicious animals do not occur. It is assumed that there is no threat or physical danger associated with the work situation. The usual safety need is for emotional security and support. Most people feel at least a partial dependence on their employer. When an employee feels insecure, threatened, or highly dependent in his or her work situation, then he or she is not concerned with social needs, esteem needs, or self actualization. Some employees are adaptable and do not feel threatened by new situations or procedures. However, a dependent or fearful individual may feel insecure when a new computer is delivered in the laboratory to replace the manual method of communication. If management is arbitrary with respect to continued employment, discrimination in promotion or to favoritism in assignments, then the work place becomes unsafe, stressful, and indeed threatening. Decreased productivity and low morale may result. However, if management has clearly defined policies that are consistently adhered to, employees become less security conscious and center on social or love needs which become motivators of behavior.

*Love Needs.* Love needs include the feeling of belonging, being a part of, being accepted by one's associates, giving and receiving friendship and love. This is dramatically illustrated by the behavior patterns of most teenagers, who adhere to the dress, language, and behavioral customs of their peer group. However, healthy adults deal first with family relationships and close knit ties. Once comfortable and secure with this group, they will turn to establish relationships with others outside the family. The absence of this support group of friends and family is keenly felt. For a child, the separation from parents and familiar surroundings for a hospital stay can be a terrifying experience.

For many people, the work setting is their social group. Here, they find fulfillment of the belonging need. The predictability of this group acceptance provides each person with support and a sense of recognition as an important group member. The belonging need expands beyond the internal person to the external with time. As an example, the group pressure at work may either inhibit productivity or facilitate productivity to meet the goals of the organization.

*Ego or Esteem Needs.* There are two facets to the level of ego or esteem need; one is internal, and the other is external. Essential is the individual's need to think well of and believe in him or herself. Esteem needs can be defined by how competent one feels to meet his or her current and future needs; by his or her perceived self-image as either a success or failure; and his or her impression as to the ability to acquire knowledge and skills for future situations.

The external aspect of ego needs are provided by others in terms of reputation, feedback from others about work or technical skills, his or her ability to receive respect or trust from others, and the continuity of respect and reputation over time. Satisfaction of ego and esteem needs may be generated in the work place or the outside environment. When a person has a "positive" or "winning" image, he or she can strive to move into the next need level.

*Self Actualization.* Self actualization or self fulfillment is an on-going continuum or cyclical set of needs to reach some internally defined personal goal. Projects are begun and completed; new projects are undertaken.

In summary, at any one point in time, a person may be fulfilling his or her social ego and self actualization needs in overlapping layers of concern. It is important to remember that "Thus man is a perpetually wanting animal. Ordinarily, the satisfaction of these wants is not altogether mutually exclusive but only tends to be. The average member of our society is most often partially satisfied and partially unsatisfied in all his/her wants."[6]

***Douglas McGregor.*** In 1960 D. McGregor published *The Human Side of Enterprise* and radically changed the mode by which people look at motivation within a work setting. Traditionally, managers have felt that:

1. "The average human being has an inherent dislike of work and will avoid it if he can.
2. Because of this basic characteristic of dislike of work, most people must be coerced, controlled, directed, threatened with punishment to get them to put forth adequate effort toward the achievement of organizational objectives.
3. The average human being prefers to be directed, wishes to avoid responsibility, has relatively little ambition, wants security above all."

McGregor called these statements Theory X and reformulated a new set of assumptions that he called Theory Y which provided an improved basis for predicting human behavior at work. The basic assumptions of Theory Y are:

1. "The expenditure of physical and mental effort in work is as natural as play or rest." (Work may be a source of satisfaction if the conditions are right.)
2. "External control and the threat of punishment are not the only means for bringing about effort toward organizational objectives. Man will exercise self-direction and self-control in the service of objectives to which he/she is committed.
3. Commitment to objectives is a function of the rewards associated with their achievement. The most significant of such rewards, e.g., the satisfaction of ego and self-actualization needs, can be direct products of effort directed toward organizational objectives.

4. The average human being learns, under proper conditions, not only to accept but to seek responsibility. Avoidance of responsibility, lack of ambition, and emphasis on security are generally consequences of experience, not inherent human characteristics.
5. The capacity to exercise a relatively high degree of imagination, ingenuity and creativity in the solution of organizational problems is widely, not narrowly, distributed in the population.
6. Under the conditions of modern industrial life, the intellectual potentialities of the average human being are only partially utilized."[7]

McGregor's study emphasized that the factors which motivate employees are very different from those that managers and teachers have long supported and enforced. Several behavioral scientists have taken Theory Y assumptions as the foundation for further applied practical research into motivation in the work place.

*Frederick Herzberg.* Organizational research with engineers and accountants was F. Herzberg's starting point. His studies have been repeated many times with other occupational groups and in other countries. Some of the other occupational groups involved have been: agricultural administrators, nurses, hospital maintenance men, professional women, lower level supervisors, military officers, scientists, housekeepers, technicians, female assemblers, teachers, Finnish foremen, and Hungarian engineers. The findings of these studies with supportive evidence from many others suggest:

1. "The factors that establish or aid motivation and job satisfaction are distinct and separate from those that produce job dissatisfaction.
2. Job satisfaction and job dissatisfaction are not just the opposites of each other as had been supposed."[8]
3. Two different human needs are involved:
   a. One drive is very basic and can come from the response to pain/hunger, in the environment. The need for food is translated to money to buy food; a way is needed to earn money, a job. Money then becomes a specific need or drive. This relates to job environment or avoidance of the pain of hunger.
   b. The other need is related to the esteem need. Man experiences emotional satisfaction and growth through achievement. This relates to the job content.
4. The growth factors that provide motivation on the job are: achievement, recognition for achievement, the work itself, responsibility, and growth or advancement.
5. The avoidance–hygiene factors that are part of the job setting are:

company policy and administration, supervision, interpersonal relationships, working conditions, salary, status, and security. If quality or quantity of these factors is high, there is no "dissatisfaction," not "satisfaction." Their presence may not motivate but their absence will cause dissatisfaction. These factors were established by asking each participant which job events had led to extreme satisfaction or extreme dissatisfaction on their part. What emerged was a "job enrichment" theory, which suggests that work should be enriched, not enlarged, to bring about more effective utilization of personnel.

This theory along with others is being tested. It takes large samples to provide reliable results because of the complex diverse nature of man.

Motivation has been defined as inducing people to act in a desired manner. People either perform of their own choice or they are persuaded to perform. Attitude, however, is the personal feeling expressed in words or behaviors. Some behavioral scientists fell that an internal stimulus moves us to be motivated. However, feelings that are expressed either verbally or in activities are a portrayal of attitudes. Others theorize that attitudes are expressions of how people feel and see themselves in terms of any given situation. A specimen control supervisor may say that a phlebotomist has a negative attitude about a patient because of observed behavior on the part of the employee that exhibits unacceptable actions. Attitudes may be vague or concrete and defined. The work setting should provide a climate that makes positive motivation and attitude development possible. Some people use personality to express what is meant about attitude. The right personality for the health-care field can be defined as a caring personality coupled with a willingness to help and do things for others. A cheerful disposition, even temper, methodical, and reliable nature are valuable assets in any setting particularly in dealing with patients. If the phlebotomist can be polite, tactful, efficient, and calm in emergencies, then the interpersonal relationships on the phlebotomy team can be pleasant and work can be performed with little friction.

### Ethics
The principles of right and wrong conduct as they apply to professional problems are the "ethics" for that profession. Professions set standards of conduct for members and expect those standards of performance to be adhered to in their work. In the health-care field, the ideal of behavior for physicians continues to be expressed in the *Hippocratic Oath,* whose text includes:

> I will prescribe regimen for the good of my patients according to my ability and my judgment and never do harm to anyone. To please none will I prescribe a deadly drug, nor give advice which may cause his/her death. Nor will I give a woman a pessary to procure abortion.

But I will preserve the purity of my life and my art. I will not cut for stone, even for patients in whom the disease is manifest; I will leave this operation to be performed by practitioners (specialists in this art). In every house where I come I will enter only for the good of my patients . . . all that may come to my knowledge in the exercise of my profession or outside of my profession or in daily commune with men, which ought not to be spread abroad, I will keep secret and never reveal.[9]

Written about 400 years before Christ, this oath is still taken by physicians around the world before entering practice. Standards of behavior are implied in the oath for each member of the health-care team. The major points are:

1. Do no harm to anyone intentionally.
2. Perform according to sound ability and good judgment.
3. Do that for which training has occurred, not more.
4. Do not become involved in anyone's care out of curiosity, only deal with those to whom assigned.
5. Facts about patients are not to be part of conversation but kept confidential.

**Florence Nightingale.** Another historical figure that had profound influence on performance standard and ethical expectations for nonphysician members of the health-care team was Florence Nightingale. In the 1850s, she practiced and wrote on hospital administration to provide reasonable care for the sick. She is credited with being the first nurse that defined not only high standards of personal behavior but wrote extensively on expectations of cleanliness and management in British hospitals. Her contributions to public health have been overshadowed by the work she did to establish the field of nursing.

**James Campbell Todd, M.D.** In 1875, at the University of Michigan in Ann Arbor, the first clinical medicine laboratory was founded. In 1908, J.C. Todd, M.D., produced a manual of *Clinical Diagnosis* which was the standard of practice for many years. This manual is now a two volume reference set of over 2000 pages with John Bernard Henry, M.D., as Editor-in-Chief. The responsibilities have grown for technical personnel in the clinical laboratory field to maintain high standards of quality control in methodology, procedure, and practices as more and more physicians realize the need for and use of diagnostic testing to improve patient care.

**The American Society for Medical Technology.** Just as physicians and nursing personnel have developed a Code of Ethics, the laboratory professionals known as Medical Technologists or Clinical Laboratory Scientists have developed a standard of performance and expressed these expectations in a code. The major theses of the code are:

1. Accuracy and reliability of laboratory test results
2. Confidentiality[10]

*The National Phlebotomy Association.* The National Phlebotomy Association has also designated responsibilities for the phlebotomist. As a newly defined subgroup in the area of providing laboratory service, the phlebotomist will:

1. Represent the Clinical Laboratory or Department of Laboratory Medicine.
2. Become knowledgeable in the behavioral sciences and apply that knowledge to human relationships with patients and fellow health-care team members.
3. Maintain accuracy, reliability, and reproducibility of results.
4. Respect the Patient's Bill of Rights.
5. Serve within the specified framework of his or her skills as defined by the hospital or laboratory standards of performance and phlebotomist job description.[11]

The phlebotomist, as in other areas of the laboratory, must continue to upgrade and maintain quality of skills. He or she must know about new techniques, new tubes, changing time constraints on tests, computer data, and changes in scientific knowledge. The phlebotomist must accept the concept that patient safety and quality care come before saving time. He or she should also be willing to ask for assistance when dealing with a difficult patient or procedure. A phlebotomist collects only those specimens ordered by the physician and the ones that he or she has been trained to collect.

In summary, ethical conduct can be expressed in routine behavior by the phlebotomist if he or she:

1. is polite to patients, regardless of the circumstances;
2. does not discuss the patient's ailments with him or her;
3. does not discuss the respective merits of the various forms of therapy;
4. never prescribes;
5. does not discuss the physician with the patient;
6. keeps appropriate records of specimen collection as described in institutional policy;
7. is alert to hazards for patient and other members of the health-care team.[11]

When considering the implications of ethical behavior, the concepts of honesty, integrity, and regard for the dignity of other human beings, continue to be the personal foundations for professional codes. Only the phlebotomist dealing with patients on a "one to one" basis knows for sure whether the work he or she performs each day is based on tenets for optimum behavior.


## APPEARANCE

One clue to a person's attitude can be general appearance and grooming. In the past, most hospitals, clinical laboratories, and physicians offices had dress codes that carefully detailed the acceptable clothing for that health-care setting. Surprisingly, today the white uniform or white laboratory coat is unacceptable in some special areas. Child Health Clinics and Children's Hospitals have decided that informal business clothing is appropriate wear when dealing with children. The white coat or smock is used to cover and protect clothing while in the technical or analytic area. However, there are clinics, hospitals, and physicians offices that still follow the more traditional dress code. The following rules generally apply to personnel who routinely interact with patients:

1. *White uniform.* The complete white uniform should be worn with white shoes. Clogs, tennis shoes, sandals, and other casual styles are not appropriate. The entire uniform and shoes should be neat and clean. It is recommended that women wear hose without seams, that jewelry be limited to rings and a wrist watch, that nails be filed short, kept clean, and without polish. Hand lotion should be available because of drying due to frequent hand washing. Women should remember to apply makeup discretely because bright or dark colors look harsh with a white uniform. Hair should be kept neatly cut, styled, and clean. Long hair which may hide the venipuncture site or get caught in laboratory equipment must be tied back. Men who wear moustaches and/or beards should keep them neat, trimmed, and clean.

2. *White smocks or tunics or jackets.* In some clinics and hospitals, phlebotomists wear white smocks, tunics, jackets, or lab coats with dark shoes and slacks. It is recommended that a light or white shirt or blouse be worn underneath. The sleeves of the smock or lab coat should be longer than the sleeves of the blouse. A dark solid colored clip on tie may be appropriate ,and comes off easily if a patient happens to grab it.

   Supervisors should remember that the rules of dress must be applied impartially to men and women on the phlebotomy team to comply with the Equal Employment Opportunity Commission rules and regulations.

## Grooming and Physical Fitness

A vital part of a nice appearance is careful attention to personal hygiene. A daily bath or shower followed by use of deodorant is recommended. Perfume or after shave lotion should be used sparingly as patients may be allergic or find some scents overpowering and distasteful. It is important to maintain good health habits because the role of a phlebotomist requires physical stamina. Good health also improves the phlebotomist's appearance, attitude, and ability to cope with stress.

The proper uniform worn with the appropriate care, good grooming and physical fitness all contribute to a good appearance. With a pleasant smile, a positive attitude, and a neat appearance, the phlebotomist is more fully prepared to deal with patients, hospital visitors, family members, and other members of the health-care team.

## MEDICOLEGAL ASPECTS

The laws governing medicine and medical ethics complement and overlap each other. For many years, even centuries, the decision of the physician or health-care professional was unquestioned. This has changed. Health-care consumers and patients have become more aware, more critical, and much more willing to sue anyone that their lawyer feels has been at fault, including phlebotomists.

In reality, the legal system in the United States has 52 systems. Each state, the District of Columbia, and the Federal Government has a separate system. The courts are places where disputes are settled by judicial decision. Both federal and state courts generally have three levels.

1. Trial courts—some have limited and some have wide jurisdiction.
2. Intermediate—are generally courts of appeal.
3. Supreme court—of each state and of the federal system will hear only specific cases.

General state courts hear more serious civil cases in which damages of over $10,000 are in suit and in criminal actions. The law can be viewed as a system of social control[12] or the law can be described as common sense influenced by political and public policy considerations. Lawyers have become advisors to health-care professionals and institutions in matters ranging from termination of treatment to approval of experimental protocols. Some lawyers specialize in hospital law or food and drug law; personal injury lawyers handle malpractice claims, and others are especially knowledgeable about Medicaid and Worker's Compensation benefits. No lawyer can master all of these areas. William J. Curran defined "health law" as a "speciality area of law and law practice related to the medical and other health fields—such as dentistry, nursing, hospital administration, and environmental law."[12]

## Legal Terminology

To grasp the legal implication of health care, some knowledge of basic terminology is important. A few major definitions follow.

- *Litigation process*—the process of legal action to determine a decision in court. Many malpractice cases are negotiated and settled out of court.
- *Plaintiff*—the claimant who brings a lawsuit or action.
- *Defendant*—the health-care provider against whom the action or lawsuit is filed.
- *Civil law*—not criminal action, the plaintiff sues for monetary damages.
- *Criminal actions*—deal with the acts or offenses against the public welfare, can lead to imprisonment.
- *Felony*—varies by state but generally is defined as public offenses where, if defendant is convicted, he or she will spend time in jail or prison.
- *Misdemeanor*—the general term for all sorts of criminal offenses not serious enough to be classified as a felony.
- *Tort*—a legal wrong in which the person who commits it is liable for damages in civil action.
- *Malpractice*—improper or unskillful care of a patient by a member of the health-care team or any professional misconduct, unreasonable lack of skill, or fidelity in professional or judiciary duties.
- *Negligence*—the omission of something that a reasonable person, guided by considerations that ordinarily regulate human affairs, would do, or as doing something that a reasonable and prudent person would not do.[12]
- *Assault*—the unjustifiable attempt to touch another person or the threat to do so in such circumstances as to cause the other to believe that it will be carried out.
- *Battery*—the unlawful beating of another or the carrying out of threatened physical harm.
- *False imprisonment*—the unjustifiable detention of a person without a legal warrant.
- *Breach of duty*—an infraction, violation or failure to perform.[12]
- *Liable*—under legal obligation, as far as damages are concerned.
- *Invasion of privacy*—the physical intrusion upon a person; the publishing of confidential information, though true, but of such objectionable or personal nature as to be offensive.[13]

*Malpractice.* The relationship between doctor and patient is, in the legal sense, a contractual one. The basic elements involved are common with other contracts. The elements of contracts are:

- *Offer*—the physician offers to provide service either by opening an office or being on a hospital staff or both. Thus he or she has made him or herself available to patients who seek care.
- *Acceptance*—the patient visits the physician for treatment of a disease or disorder and may agree to accept medical care.
- *Consideration*—the patient accepts treatment and pays for the care provided by the physician.[13]

By completing these steps, there is a contract which implies obligations on the part of *both* the physician and the patient. The physician is obligated to provide medical care to the patient if he or she follows directions and pays for the service. There is even a question about the length of grace period in terms of payment. Also, the patient generally has to refuse treatment before the physician is legally freed from his or her obligation. By agreeing to provide service, the physician is required to provide a standard of care.

If the physician is a pathologist and medical director of a medical clinical laboratory, in most cases he or she is responsible under the law for the standard of care and performance of the laboratory staff. Therefore, a breach of standard on the part of a phlebotomist would generally be a litigation involving the pathologist.

The trend toward medical malpractice is not as new as most people seem to believe. The first case was reported in London in the 1300s. In the 1850s, Abraham Lincoln tried and won three medical malpractice cases before he was elected President.[14] It is estimated that 5 to 10 percent of the physicians in the United States are involved in medical malpractice lawsuits, i.e., negligence cases. Malpractice, in the usual sense, implies that the health-care provider did something wrong; it usually involves improper or unskilled care where the practitioner has not exercised judgment or performed to the expected standard of care.

Physicians, however, do not guarantee cures, only treatment or therapy. The patient bringing the lawsuit (plaintiff) must have been injured or damaged by the health-care professional's breach of duty (failure to use standard of care). Damage or injury may be either physical, mental, or financial.

If the patient requires treatment that is of potential risk, the physician must explain risks and alternatives prior to asking the patient to sign an "Informed Consent Form." This form is required for surgical, experimental, or other invasive procedures. The signed form is not valid unless the patient has received the necessary instructions first. This is one reason the phlebotomist should state in simple terms what the procedure for blood collection will be. Under the law, there are special rules for children and unconscious adults.

It is very difficult for a patient to win a medical malpractice case. One of the most difficult aspects for the patient is the expert witness. To win the case, the patient's expert witness must be willing to testify in court that the defendant health-care professional was negligent, i.e., that he or she did not provide the standard of care that other physicians of that speciality in that community would provide.[12] In the *Small* v. *Howard* case in 1880, the court ruled that a village practitioner would be required to have only knowledge and skills of other practitioners in "similar localities." This rule of community standard held until *Brune* v. *Belinoff* in which the court held that all specialists in anesthesiology should be aware of advanced practices of their profession regardless of location.[13]

Medical records are vital. A phlebotomist or any other member of the health-care team cannot be expected to remember a patient from whom blood was drawn 3 to 4 years ago. The medical records must be neat, legible, and accurate. They are extremely important if a medical malpractice case goes to court. It is important to remember that many cases are not in the literature because often the health-care institution or health-care provider negotiates and settles out of court.

The following are actual cases that are of interest for laboratorians:

1. *Requests by police*

   Nurses, technologists, and phlebotomists are concerned about drawing a blood sample when requested by police on an unconscious patient or lacking the patient's consent. The United States Supreme Court ruled in *Schmerber* v. *State of California* that tests performed on a blood sample drawn by a physician in a hospital from a person arrested by the police were admissible in a court action.[4] This may vary by state.

2. *Laboratory report case*

   A patient who was pregnant for the first time had her blood typed in January, 1971. The report sent to her physician was that her blood type was A positive. The patient gave birth to her second child on June 29, 1977. The child was brain damaged with paralysis on the right side of the body as a result of hemolytic blood disease of the newborn. The laboratory records in 1971 and 1977 showed the mother's blood type to be O negative. In a malpractice suit, the parents charged that the physician's and his employees' negligence caused the child's injuries. The physician, who was chief of the laboratory when the blood test was performed, was found liable, as was the phlebotomist. *Lazernick* v. *General Hospital of Monroe County* (PA 1977).[15]

3. *Respondeat Superior or vicarious liability*

   The doctrine of *respondeat superior* is applied to employees. Even though the employer is liable for the employee, both can and generally will be sued. The plaintiff's lawyers generally go after the employer because of the possibility of a larger settlement. However, employers may be cleared leaving the employee to stand or fall alone. In the mind of some professionals, the "deep pockets" concept tends to minimize the risk for laboratory employees. Generally, organizations and individuals best able to pay are the most likely candidates for suit. Job descriptions that commonly define laboratorians' duties as administrative and procedural rather than judgmental have kept technicians, technologists, and phlebotomists at low legal exposure levels.[16]

4. *Proper technique is vital*

A malpractice suit was filed against a physician for negligence in drawing a blood sample. The patient claimed that the physician damaged the radial nerve of the right wrist by failing to use a sterile needle for blood specimen collection. The site of venipuncture became swollen, tender, and inflamed. The patient testified that the needle was laid near a used tongue depressor. The same needle was used for several attempts to redraw. The patient, after retrial, was awarded monetary damages. *McCormick* v. *Auret* (GA 1980).[14]

5. *Proper use of equipment*

A patient was admitted for treatment of pneumonia. On the second day, the patient complained of cold and numbness in his right hand. On the fourth day, a vascular surgeon examined the hand and ordered 4000 units of heparin in hopes of restoring blood flow. The hand had to be amputated. In court, the expert witness testified that a blood pressure cuff had been left on for an extended period. He was awarded $40,000. *Walton* v. *Providence Hospital.*[13]

6. *Consent to treatment*

The U.S. District Court for the Southern District of Texas upheld a state judge in ordering temporary removal of an infant from her parent's custody to that of a child welfare unit and empowering the unit to provide necessary emergency medical treatment. The parents, who were Jehovah's Witnesses, refused to consent to a needed blood transfusion because of the Rh negative factor in their child's blood. The court said that the parents could not choose to make martyrs of their children. *Lacy* v. *Judge Robert Lowry.* Harris County Hospital district.[17]

## Malpractice Insurance

Often, the health-care staff in the hospital or clinic laboratory are part of a blanket malpractice insurance policy. However, if the phlebotomist is employed by a pathologist who has a contract with an institution or owns a clinic, the staff may be protected by the pathologist's malpractice insurance policy. "Medical malpractice claims and awards continue to grow in number and dollar amounts. This [trend] appears unlikely to change for a variety of reasons, including the geometric growth rate of newer technologies for diagnosis and treatment."[14]

Malpractice insurance rates for pathologists are generally the lowest premiums charged because of their low risk level. At the bench and administrative levels, laboratories have rarely been named in malpractice suits. In the five cases settled between 1975 and 1978 against laboratory technical employees, claims averaged less than $10,000. Part of the reason for so few cases is that under the legal concept of respondeat superior, responsibility for wrongful acts of the employee – agent – servant rests on the employer principal – master. Also, another reason for not being named in a suit is the "deep pocket" concept. The phlebotomist with less money or no insurance in the past has not been a target for suit. However, the advances in technology and increased complexity of health care has increased legal exposure for allied health professionals. Often, laboratorians feel safe from legal responsibilities because of limited interaction with patients. However, the phlebotomist and any other staff member that routinely deal with the public, in patient – health provider relationships, are indeed liable. Therefore, each individual should examine the possibility of malpractice suits and the need for malpractice insurance from a personal standpoint.[16]

If the phlebotomist decides to purchase malpractice insurance, there are several factors that should be carefully considered.

1. Is adequate dollar value coverage provided? Recent suits have $1,000,000 damages against physicians.
2. What are the limitations of coverage?
3. What are the procedures that must be followed for the policy to provide coverage? Some state that divulging the amount of coverage or the fact that he or she is covered voids the policy.
4. The phlebotomist should not assume that the lawyers representing the hospital, laboratory, or clinic will have his or her best interests at heart. The attorney's first obligation is to serve those who have hired him or her. There have been cases in which the hospital was cleared of all charges but the allied health professional was held liable for damages. For the phlebotomist, if an adult patient seems alert and does not object to the blood specimen collection then consent is implied. Proceeding without consent may give rise to assault and battery, as well as civil suits.

With the purchase of malpractice professional liability insurance, the attorney's fee and court costs usually are covered. Some of the professional organizations offer professional liability insurance at a reasonable or reduced rate. With the advent of organ transplantations, renal dialysis, and hyperbaric care, the avenues of liability are widened. A genuine concern for others and careful attention to technique are good investments of the phlebotomist's time. A record of continuing education courses, seminars, workshops, or academic credits should be a part of each phlebotomist's personal file.

## PROFESSIONAL ORGANIZATIONS

Two national organizations that recognize the phlebotomist as a definitive and vital part of the health-care team are:

1. *The American Society for Medical Technology (ASMT)*—has recognized medical laboratory personnel for 50 years. There are several types of memberships available depending on the education and experience of the individual. Two types of memberships are applicable.
   a. *Active Member*—medical technologist requires a baccalaureate or graduate degree in medical technology; or related field; licensure; certification; five years of experience; or completion of an accredited educational program.
   b. *Associate Member*—medical technician requires an associate degree in medical technology; or a baccalaureate in education with a minor in science; and an active interest in the goals and objectives of ASMT.[10]
   It is anticipated that there will be a certifying examination offered by National Certifying Agency (NCA) for phlebotomists in the near future. Currently, most phlebotomists are joining ASMT as associate members as part of the Phlebotomy section.
2. *The National Phlebotomy Association*—was established in 1978 to recognize the phlebotomist as a distinctive and identifiable part of the allied health team.
   a. *Active*
      i. Grandfather Clause requires 3 years of experience as a phlebotomist prior to 1978. The phlebotomist can be considered active if 60 percent or more of the work performed includes venipuncture and skin puncture blood collection.
      ii. Less than 3 years of experience prior to 1978. Must successfully complete a training program that includes at least 48 hours of classroom work, a supervised clinical experience and a passing grade on a certifying examination offered by the National Phlebotomy Association.
   b. *Nonactive Phlebotomist*
   In order to take the phlebotomy examination, the person who has not worked for 12 months or more, or one with less than 3 years of experience should:
      i. attend enough lectures, workshops, conferences to receive 3.6 Continuing Education Units (CEU) per 12-month period.

   ii. obtain 4.7 CEU to take the phlebotomy examination.
c. *Senior Phlebotomist*
A phlebotomist with 10 or more years of experience in the field. Proof of
employment and a letter of recommendation must be submitted.[11]


# DEALING WITH STRESS

Stress is very prevalent in the work place. In studies funded by the United
States Department of Labor, it was reported that nonphysician laboratory
personnel ranked third in terms of stress level experienced in the work
place. Because of rapid technologic progress, personnel have been forced
to make rapid behavioral adjustments to a faster paced and more pres-
sured life, which tends to induce stress.
   Figure 8-4 shows the possible daily interactions that occur to the phlebotomist and also the patient in a health-care setting.
   Some people prefer to cope with the stress of illness by retreating from
personal interaction. In the clinic or hospital setting, this is not possible.
Thus, stress for health-care professionals and patients can increase. What is
stress? Usually, it is defined by physiologic changes such as:

1. elevated blood pressure
2. increased heart rate
3. increased breath rate
4. increased body metabolism
5. increased blood flow to muscles

   When there is constant stress, chronic high blood pressure can result.
This is significant because it is a predisposing factor to heart attack and
stroke. These diseases of the heart and brain account for more than 50 percent of the deaths each year in the United States.[18]
   Stress may happen because of constant change with little escape from
it. Too often, the trauma associated with change is overlooked. For the
phlebotomist, the change may be a shift in work hours, the route covered,
the people one works with, the supervisor, and/or new techniques and policies.
   Hans Selye, in *The Stress of Life,* discusses what stress can be to the
human condition. Selye said "Stress is not even necessarily bad for you; it is
also the spice of life, for any emotion, any activity causes stress." A certain
level of stress pushes people to achieve, to win, and to compete. However,
too much may incapacitate or make a person ill. Selye's research into the
impact of stress on the body led him to conclude that rest can *almost* restore
the body to the prior level of fitness. Like a piece of elastic pulled too tight
for too long, when released it does not quite return to the original shape.
   Selye also concluded that exposure to stress does not necessarily make

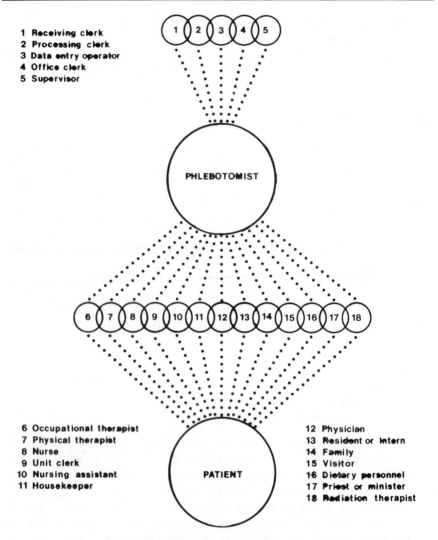

1 Receiving clerk
2 Processing clerk
3 Data entry operator
4 Office clerk
5 Supervisor

PHLEBOTOMIST

6 Occupational therapist
7 Physical therapist
8 Nurse
9 Unit clerk
10 Nursing assistant
11 Housekeeper

12 Physician
13 Resident or Intern
14 Family
15 Visitor
16 Dietary personnel
17 Priest or minister
18 Radiation therapist

PATIENT

**Figure 8-4.** Interaction pathways.

it easier to withstand greater stress. It may make the body even more vulnerable. "Wear and tear" on the body caused by stress may lead to premature aging.[19]

Bettina Martin in a lecture, "Dealing With Stress and Making It Work for You," suggested some rules for low stress living.

1. Make time your ally, not your master.
2. Associate mostly with gentle people who affirm your personhood.
3. Learn and practice the skill of deep relaxation.
4. Use aerobic exercise to improve health.

5. Engage in satisfying, meaningful work.
6. Don't let your work dominate your entire life.
7. Find some time in every day for complete privacy.
8. Open yourself up to new experiences. Find self-renewing opportunities.
9. Read interesting books and articles to freshen your ideas and broaden your point of view.
10. Don't bite off more than you can chew.
11. Seek rewarding experiences in all dimensions of living.
12. Surround yourself with cues that affirm positive thoughts and positive approaches to life and that remind you to relax and unwind occasionally.[20]

Keith Schnert, M.D., has some additional coping ideas in his book *Stress/Unstress*. He suggested that by using visualization (see a favorite place vividly in the mind), relaxation and fun the level of stress can be dramatically reduced. Also, each person should sing in the shower, do bend and stretch exercises, and take time to relax.[21] By using appropriate techniques to deal with stress, doing some reasonable planning, and being aware of the importance of time management, the phlebotomist can cope more successfully with the stress of working as part of the health-care team. In the work setting, knowing the job skills to perform the techniques and procedures well, having good interpersonal relationships, and understanding more about human behavior can aid the phlebotomist in approaching each day more positively and productively.

## STUDY QUESTIONS

1. In identifying the alert adult in-patient, what are the major steps for the phlebotomist to follow?
2. After an out-patient has had a venipuncture performed, what techniques should the phlebotomist follow before dismissing the patient?
3. List the diseases that disqualify a blood donor.
4. List seven of the major topics in the "Patient's Bill of Rights" that are important for the phlebotomist to remember.
5. List the four major contributors to the study of human behavior and motivation.
6. Outline Maslow's hierarchy of human needs.
7. Outline McGregor's Theory X.
8. Outline McGregor's Theory Y.
9. What is the major difference between civil and criminal law?
10. Most suits in malpractice cases are based on the difference between actual performance and expected performance in the health-care setting. How is the expected performance usually expressed?

# REFERENCES

1. Erikson EH: Childhood and Society, 2nd ed. New York, Norton, 1963.
2. Widmann FK (ed): Technical Manual of the American Association of Blood Banks. American Association of Blood Banks, 1981.
3. Patient's Bill of Rights, American Hospital Association, 1973.
4. Ford CW, Morgan MK (eds): Teaching in the Health Professions, St. Louis, Mosby, 1978.
5. Roethlisberger FJ: Management and Morale, Cambridge, Massachusetts, Harvard University Press, 1956.
6. Maslow AH: Motivation and Personality, 2nd ed. New York, Harper & Row, 1970.
7. McGregor D: The Human Side of Enterprise, New York McGraw-Hill, 1960.
8. Hertzberg F: One more time: How do you motivate employees? Harvard Business Review, Trustees of Harvard University, 1968.
9. Duncan AS, Dunstan GR, Welbourne RB (eds): Dictionary of Medical Ethics, New Rev Ed. New York, Crossroad Publishing, 1981.
10. American Society for Medical Technology, Passport to Success (Brochure).
11. National Phlebotomy Association, Guidelines, 1980.
12. Curran WJ: Titles in the medico legal field: A proposal for reform. Amer J Law Medicine 1:10, 1975.
13. Creighton H: Law Every Nurse Should Know, 4th ed. Philadelphia, Saunders, 1981.
14. Glasscock D: Legal Implications of Laboratory Medicine (Lecture Notes), July 15, 1981.
15. Lazernick v General Hospital of Monroe County (PA-1977).
16. Zeiler WB: How your lab can minimize malpractice risks. Medical Laboratory Observer, May, 1982.
17. Lacy v Judge Robert Lowry, Harris County Hospital District, et al., U.S.D.T. No. 74-H-124, March 16, 1977.
18. Benson H: Your innate asset for combating stress. Harvard Business Review #74402, July–August, 1974.
19. Selye H: The Stress of Life, 2nd ed. New York, McGraw-Hill, 1978.
20. Martin BG: Dealing With Stress and Making It Work For You. Lecture at a meeting of American Society of Clinical Pathologists.
21. Sehnert KW: Stress–Unstress, Minneapolis, Augsburg Press, 1981.

# CHAPTER 9

# Quality Control and Safety in Blood Collection

Kathleen Becan-McBride

Clinical laboratory test results are increasingly used by physicians for diagnosis and treatment of their patients. Thus, every step in the formulation of these results must be of superlative quality. Clinical laboratories are responsible for the methodology that assures reliable, accurate test results. The method used to assure reliable, accurate data is referred to as quality control. Quality control plays a major part in the laboratory in (1) patient preparation and specimen collection, (2) specimen transportation and processing, (3) instrumental and technical performance of clinical laboratory assays, (4) laboratory safety, and (5) in-service training and education of laboratorians and other health-care professionals.

The quality control officer, clinical laboratory supervisor, and/or laboratory director usually regulate the quality control program in the clinical laboratory. The size of the laboratory and number of staff generally indicate who handles the quality control policies and tasks.

All laboratory personnel must follow all quality control policies and procedures to assure quality patient care. Because specimen collection is the first step in the process of acquiring quality results, the phlebotomist must provide the laboratory with perfect specimens.

## COLLECTION PROCEDURES TO INSURE QUALITY

In order to obtain perfect specimens, first the patient and the specimen container must be prepared. If the patient is not adequately prepared, the laboratory procedures and instrumentation cannot compensate for the shortcomings. Thus, the clinical laboratory must provide the nursing staff with a floor book (Table 9-1) that describes preparation of the patient and special handling of patient's specimens. The phlebotomist should be aware of the protocol that is necessary to prepare patients and specimen containers for laboratory assays in order to instruct the nursing staff in this capacity, and therefore, lead to quality specimen collection. Thus, a monthly review of the laboratory's collection procedures and policies is recommended to reduce collection errors and hopefully lead to perfect specimen collection. Examples of the types of collection procedures that the phlebotomist should review include:

1. Collection of blood specimens by skin puncture
2. Isolation techniques
3. Microcollection techniques on newborns
4. Capillary blood gases
5. Collection of blood specimens by fingerstick
6. Intensive care blood collections
7. Pediatric blood collection techniques
8. Collection of specimens for intravenous glucose tolerance tests
9. Collection of biohazardous specimens
10. Inability to collect blood specimen
11. Patient identification

Also, the phlebotomist should have access to a pocket-sized collection booklet that contains the same information as in the floor book (i.e., laboratory test, laboratory section in which procedure is performed, required collection container, amount of required sample, preservatives for sample handling).

Some examples of patient preparation and specimen container preparation include:

1. The patient must ingest at least 300 g of carbohydrates daily for at least 3 days prior to glucose tolerance test.
2. The patient must be fasting for 12 to 16 hours before a glucose analysis.
3. The mechanics of the glucose tolerance test should be explained to the patient before the test so that he or she will understand the reason for fasting prior to the test. The fasting blood specimen is collected in the morning rather than at a random collection time to avoid the following laboratory test results:
   a. the effects of exercise,
   b. the effects of changes in posture, and
   c. the effects of diurnal variation.
4. A fasting specimen is desirable for triglyceride and cholesterol analysis.

**TABLE 9-1. SAMPLE PAGE FROM FLOOR BOOK: TEST INFORMATION**

| Test | Sample Fluid | Minimum Volume (ml) | Special Handling | Reference Range | Days Available | Usual Reporting Time |
|---|---|---|---|---|---|---|
| Blood gases | WB (heparin) | 1 | Arterial blood collected in a heparinized syringe. Transport on ice. | pH: 7.35–7.45 $Po_2$: 88–108 mm Hg $Pco_2$: 35–45 mm Hg | All (all) | 10 min |
| Bromide | S | 4 | | Th: 1–2 mg/ml | M-F (9 AM) | 8 hours |
| Bromsulfaphalein clearance | S | 3 | Collect 45 min after administration of dye | <7% retention | M-F (9 AM) | 8 hours |
| Calcium, ionized | S | 2 | Collect on ice. Submit immediately | 2.20–2.60 mEq/liter | M-F (9 AM) | 8 hours |
| Calcium total | S | 2 | | 8.5–10.5 mg/dl | All (all) | 8 hours |
| | U | 10 | 24 hours timed specimen Add 10 ml conc. HCl to bottle prior to collection | 40–220 mg/24 hours | All (9 AM) | 8 hours |
| Carbamazepine | S | 1 | | Th: 2–12 µg/ml | M-F (9 AM, 5 PM) | 8 hours |
| Carbon dioxide content | S | 2 | | 24–32 mEq/liter | All (all) | 4 hours |
| Carbon monoxide | U | 0.5 | CALL PATHOLOGIST | | | |
| | P (oxalate) | 1 | Heparinized samples are only stable for up to 2 hours | Nonsmokers: 0.5–2% saturation Smokers: 9% saturation | M-F (9 AM, 5 PM) | 4 hours |
| Carotene | S | 5 | | 50–200 µg/dl | M (9 AM) | 8 hours |
| Catecholamines, total | U | 50 | 24 hour timed specimen. Add 10 ml conc. HCl to bottle prior to collection | 32–103 µg/24 hours | Th (9 AM) | 8 hours |

*(From Hermann Hospital Clinical Laboratories, with permission.)*

5. Ten milliliters of concentrated hydrochloric acid (HCl) must be added to a 24-hour urine collection container prior to collection in order to preserve the clinical constituents to be analyzed in the laboratory.

## Anticoagulants and Preservatives: Quality Assurance

As discussed in Chapter 3, the phlebotomist uses various anticoagulants and preservatives in the collection of blood specimens. These tubes containing anticoagulants must be inverted promptly after blood is drawn to assure mixture of the anticoagulant and blood and thus provide quality assurance of a perfectly collected specimen. As reviewed in Chapter 5, when several evacuated tubes of blood are collected on a patient, tubes containing anticoagulants should be filled last so that proper inversion can occur and carry over of anticoagulants to clotted tubes will not occur.

In order to assure quality, the anticoagulants and preservatives should meet the requirements established by the National Committee for Clinical Laboratory Standards.[1] The manufacturer of the anticoagulants and preservatives must provide the shelf-life of these additives on the packages so that the user will know how long these additives are effective. In addition, for blood collection tubes, the manufacturers must test and verify draw and fill accuracy until the stated expiration date. The phlebotomist should be cognizant of expiration dates on any item used in specimen collection.

In addition, quality can only be obtained in specimen collection with fresh specimens. If the blood specimen is not to be run immediately, the phlebotomist must make certain that it is stored properly until the test is run. For example, if the specimen is to be shipped to a reference laboratory, the phlebotomist should review the laboratory procedure on the "Handling of Specimen for Reference Laboratory Work" (Table 9-2) to prepare the specimen in the proper manner and maintain a suitable specimen for the laboratory test. Breakage and leakage may also result during shipping if the specimen is not packaged properly.

## Requirements for a Quality Specimen

The requirements for a quality specimen include the following:

1. The patient is prepared properly and drug interference is avoided, if possible.
2. The correct specimens are collected from the correct patients with the proper labeling. Because it is the policy of most clinical laboratories to discard specimens that are unlabeled or labeled incorrectly, the phlebotomist must abide by the written laboratory policy describing acceptable identification of specimens to insure perfect specimen collection. The potential errors in after-the-fact reidentification of a specimen by floor personnel can be extremely detrimental to the patient in question and must be avoided. (Refer to Chapter 4 for identification and labeling procedures.)

**TABLE 9-2. HANDLING OF SAMPLES FOR REFERENCE LABORATORY WORK**

**Principle**

Specimen Control will have responsibility for the receipt, record-keeping, and dispatch of all clinical specimens to be sent to reference laboratories. This will insure adequate centralized control over the entire process from specimen collection to reporting.

**Procedure**

1. All specimens for reference laboratories will be accumulated in a refrigerator/freezer in the Specimen Control Laboratory. After 3:30 PM, all specimens will be processed and accumulated in the Chemistry Laboratory; these specimens are then retrieved by Specimen Control the following morning. Specimens will be dispatched to each reference laboratory at least once daily, Monday through Friday. Specimens requiring special handling must receive immediate attention.

2. As each sample is processed the following information will be entered on the request slip. "Send to _____ " (name of reference laboratory), date sent and technologist's initials.

3. A log book will be immediately available if any questions should arise concerning sample collection or status. The log book will contain the date the specimen was sent, the patient's name, date of collection, unit number, room number, the test requested, the particular reference laboratory, test results, and the date the results were received.

4. An alphabetical file (by patient's last name) will be kept in Specimen Control on work pending. The original request slip will remain in this file until results are received from the reference laboratory.

5. When reports are received from the reference laboratory, the results and date received will be entered on the original request slip, which is then processed according to usual protocol. Results and the date they were received will also be entered in the log book. Reference laboratory original reports will be filed in a separate file alphabetically by patient's name.

6. All reports must be reviewed by the appropriate doctorate staff member.

7. All physicians' copies must be mailed by the supervisor or assistant supervisor of Specimen Control to the physician whose name appears on the request slip.

8. Specimen Control will have the responsibility for handling the billing documents for all reference laboratory work. Each billing document will be labeled with the proper eight digit service code number for each test ordered. Rare tests will be assigned the miscellaneous service code number of 40199993 with a description of the test written in. The catalog cost of the test must also be written in. The service code number for handling of a specimen is 40199977. This code number must appear on every reference laboratory test billing document either alone or accompanied by another service code number.

9. All invoices from reference laboratories will be checked against the log book and, as necessary, other file documents to verify that all reports have been received and recorded by the Laboratory Medicine or Pathology Department and that all charges are legitimate.

10. Supportive documents for all reference laboratory work will be kept in alphabetical file for 2 years in Specimen Control.

11. A master file of all reference procedures on the approved list will be kept in Specimen Control. These will be filed alphabetically by test name and will contain all needed information concerning each procedure such as the reference lab performing procedure, sample required, special handling of sample, cost and approximate turnaround time of procedure.

**Notes**

1. All requests for clinical procedures not performed in the Department of Pathology and Laboratory Medicine must be submitted to Specimen Control with the appropriate specimens, request slips, and billing documents. Pathology will not handle the reporting of or billing for any procedures unless this protocol is followed.

2. Samples will be sent only to the reference laboratory designated for the particular test. Recommendations for permanent addition to or changes of this list must be submitted to the Chairman, Department of Pathology and Laboratory Medicine. For the rare tests which are not included on the list of approved reference laboratories, a laboratory may be designated on an emergency basis by the Administrative Laboratory Manager or Assistant Laboratory Manager after consultation with the appropriate doctorate staff.

*(From Hermann Hospital Clinical Laboratories, with permission.)*

3. The correct anticoagulants and/or preservatives are used with the sufficient amount collected. (See Chapter 3 on Anticoagulants and Preservatives.)

4. The specimens are not hemolyzed.

5. The fasting specimens are collected in a timely fashion and are actually fasting samples.

6. Timed specimens are correctly timed and documented.

7. Specimens are transported to the clinical laboratory in a timely fashion to maintain freshness.

In order to conform to these requirements, the phlebotomist should review the clinical laboratory's procedures to identify the designated delivery times (Table 9-3) for each laboratory procedure. If the laboratory does not have designated delivery times for specimens, the phlebotomist may wish to suggest to his or her laboratory supervisor that such a system would insure fresh specimens, and thus, high quality laboratory results. A list of the specimens that are delivered after the designated time limits should be maintained in the specimen collection area. Such a list can usually help detect the source of the problem so that quality assurance can be maintained in the specimen control section. The list reveals how late and the number of specimens that were delivered after the allowable limits. The supervisor of specimen control usually decides whether the late specimen should be discarded and recollected.

**TABLE 9-3. EXAMPLES OF DESIGNATED DELIVERY TIMES FOR LABORATORY SPECIMENS**

| | |
|---|---|
| *Clinical microbiology* | |
| Routine bacterial culture | |
| Swab with holding medium | 90 min |
| Swab without holding medium | 20 min |
| Body fluids | 40 min |
| *Parasitology* | |
| Feces for amoeba identification | Immediately |
| *Clinical chemistry* | |
| Glucose | 20 min |
| Enzymes | 30 min |
| $Na^+$, $K^+$, $Cl^-$, $HCO_3$ (electrolytes) | 30 min |
| Chemical profile | 45 min |
| *Coagulation* | |
| Prothrombin time (PT) | 45 min |
| Partial thromboplastin time (PTT) | 45 min |
| Clotting time | Immediately |
| *Urinalysis/clinical microscopy* | |
| Routine urinalysis | 90 min |

In addition to insuring that the delivery times for specimens are maintained, the phlebotomist and the nursing staff should be aware of the test procedures that must be scheduled with the specimen control section in the laboratory. For example, to insure that enough phlebotomists are available for glucose tolerance tests, it is advisable to have the glucose tolerance test scheduled with specimen control at least 24 hours prior to the test. The persons scheduling the test should be entered into a glucose tolerance test log book. A cutoff number of scheduled glucose tolerance tests should be determined for the specimen control section to insure that the phlebotomists will be able to obtain every specimen at the proper time. Other frequently encountered laboratory assays that must be scheduled in advance include blood specimens drawn for drug monitoring. This scheduling process is another means to assure quality specimen collection.

### Number of Blood Collection Attempts

Another way the specimen control section of the laboratory can provide quality assurance to the patients is by logging the number of unsuccessful collection attempts. If the phlebotomist has had consecutively unsuccessful attempts to draw blood from different patients, the supervisor and phlebotomist will know that the problem in blood collection must be identified and solved to avoid future unsuccessful attempts. Most clinical laboratories have a written procedure on the "Inability to Draw Specimens" (Table 9-4) which describes the steps that should be taken by the phlebotomist in (a) unsuccessful collection attempts, b) patient unavailability, and (c) patient refusal.

Also, a log should be kept on the number of times that blood has been collected from pediatric and newborn patients (Fig. 9-1). Due to their blood volume, it is best to collect the minimum required amount of blood for each laboratory assay to avoid significant blood loss during their hospital stay. Each laboratory should have a table of maximum amounts of blood that can be drawn on these patients, as shown in Table 9-5. The log book provides a check on the amount of blood that has been drawn from these patients to avoid problems in significant blood loss.

### Quality Control in the Collection of Blood Cultures

As discussed in Chapter 5, the phlebotomist's main concern when obtaining a blood culture specimen is to prevent contamination of the blood culture by skin organisms. The quality control procedures that should be adhered to by the phlebotomist in order to prevent contamination include:

1. The venipuncture site should not be touched after it has been prepared for needle insertion.
2. Unsterile gauze should not be put over the venipuncture site until after blood is drawn.

**TABLE 9-4. INABILITY TO DRAW SPECIMENS**

1. A maximum of two laboratory employees will attempt to obtain blood from a patient.
2. Any unsuccessful attempt to obtain blood *must* be documented.
3. All documentation is to be made on the main part of the requisition, *not* on the tear portion.
4. Patient unavailable
   a. If you are unable to obtain blood when requested because a patient is unavailable (gone to x-ray or surgery, out of room, etc.), hold these slips until you have completed all other patients on that nursing unit. Check the patient's room again before leaving unit.
   b. If patient is still unavailable, notify the primary nurse. Leave the slip(s) at the desk with the following information:
      i. reason patient unavailable
      ii. time and initials of collector/technologist
      iii. name or nurse notified
      The patient will then be drawn on the next scheduled run.
5. Patient refused
   If patient refuses to be drawn, notify the primary nurse. Leave the slips at the unit desk with the following information:
   a. patient refused
   b. time and initials of collector/technologist
   c. name of nurse notified
6. Patient missed
   a. If at any time the person collecting blood is unable to obtain the blood, he or she should check to see if there is another collector/technologist to help.
   b. If no other laboratory employee is available, notify the patient's nurse that the patient was missed and that another person from the laboratory will try on the next run unless nurse requests attempt to be made sooner. Leave the slips at the desk with the following information:
      i. patient missed
      ii. time, initials of collector/technologist
      iii. name of nurse notified
   c. Upon returning to the laboratory, notify the Specimen Control Laboratory. A collector will then attempt to obtain the specimen at the next collection run unless otherwise requested.
   d. If the second person is unable to obtain the specimen, a nurse is again notified and the above information is again documented on the requisition. At this time request that a physician draw the blood.

| | |
|---|---|
| Supervisor | Laboratory Director |

*(From Hermann Hospital Clinical Laboratories, with permission.)*

3. The requisition must show the date and time of the blood culture collection and the initials of the phlebotomist who collected it.

Sometimes, even with all of the precautions in blood culture collection, contamination occurs. To determine the rate and possible source of blood culture contamination, the clinical microbiology section may maintain a written or computer log to tabulate negative and positive culture results and contaminated specimens. This log can detect the contamination rate of blood cultures and the particular shift when the blood culture was col-

Week _1_    Month _March_    Year _1984_
Collection Log on Pediatric and Newborn Patients

| Date | Patient | Age | Patient Number | Floor | Test Requested | Amount Collected |
|---|---|---|---|---|---|---|
| 3-4-84 | Rubinoff, Baby | 4 days | 1650421 | NB Nur | SMAC 20 | 3 microtainers |
| 3-4-84 | Gustafson, H. | 5 yrs | 177482 | 6B | electrolytes | 2 × 250 μl |
| 3-4-84 | Benson, J. | 12 mo | 185621 | 6B | Hb & Hct | 2 × 20 μl |

**Figure 9-1.** Blood collections on pediatric and newborn patients. *(Courtesy of Hermann Hospital Clinical Laboratory.)*

lected. Thus, high contamination rates may be traced to an individual with poor collection practices, such as inadequate cleansing of the venipuncture area.

## Quality Control and Preventive Maintenance on Specimen Control Instruments

The phlebotomist should be aware that quality control and preventive maintenance occurs on certain instruments and equipment in the specimen control section. For example, as shown in Table 9-6, the thermometers are

**TABLE 9-5. MAXIMUM AMOUNTS OF BLOOD TO BE DRAWN ON PATIENTS UNDER 14 YEARS**

| Pounds | kg (Approx) | Maximum Amount to be Drawn at Any One Time (ml) | Maximum Amount of Blood (Cumulative) During a Given Hospital Stay (1 month or under) (ml) |
|---|---|---|---|
| 6–8 | 2.7–3.6 | 2.5 | 23 |
| 8–10 | 3.6–4.5 | 3.5 | 30 |
| 10–15 | 4.5–6.8 | 5 | 40 |
| 16–20 | 7.3–9.1 | 10 | 60 |
| 21–25 | 9.5–11.4 | 10 | 70 |
| 26–30 | 11.8–13.6 | 10 | 80 |
| 31–35 | 14.1–15.9 | 10 | 100 |
| 36–40 | 16.4–18.2 | 10 | 130 |
| 41–45 | 18.6–20.5 | 20 | 140 |
| 46–50 | 20.9–22.7 | 20 | 160 |
| 51–55 | 23.2–25.0 | 20 | 180 |
| 56–60 | 25.5–27.3 | 20 | 200 |
| 61–65 | 27.7–29.5 | 25 | 220 |
| 66–70 | 30.0–31.8 | 30 | 240 |
| 71–75 | 32.3–34.1 | 30 | 250 |
| 76–80 | 34.5–36.4 | 30 | 270 |
| 81–85 | 36.8–38.6 | 30 | 290 |
| 86–90 | 39.1–40.9 | 30 | 310 |
| 91–95 | 41.4–43.2 | 30 | 330 |
| 96–100 | 43.6–45.5 | 30 | 350 |

*(From Hermann Hospital Clinical Laboratories, with permission.)*

**TABLE 9-6. QUALITY CONTROL AND PREVENTIVE MAINTENANCE OF THERMOMETERS**

**Standards to be Achieved and Maintained**

Prior to placing in service, all thermometers must meet the following specifications:

| Location | Usual Temperature Range | Allowable Deviation from NBS Standard |
|---|---|---|
| Refrigerators | 0 to 6°C | 1°C |
| Freezers | −5 to −20°C | 2°C |
| Incubators | 20 to 40°C | 1°C |
| Heat blocks | above 100°C | 2°C |

Thermometers which fail to meet requirements cannot be used and should be referred to the Supervisor for return to manufacturer.

**Calibration Procedure**

1. Thermometers should be tested against an NBS certified thermometer within or near the temperature ranges intended for use. Refrigerator thermometers should be calibrated near 0°C, freezers near −10°C, and so on. Both the standard thermometer and thermometer being tested should be held in water, mineral oil, or other suitable fluid to avoid rapid changes in temperature while reading.
2. Recalibration is required (a) when a thermometer calibrated in one temperature range is to be used in another temperature range, (b) when a thermometer is suspected to be damaged (dropping or other accidents), and (c) on an annual basis to assure continued accuracy.
3. Each thermometer will be given a number and this number will be recorded in a quality control book and kept in the office of the quality control coordinator. This book must be signed out and returned by supervisors to record calibration data each time new thermometers are installed in service.

Calibrated thermometers may be obtained from the Quality Control coordinator in case of an emergency need.

**Quality Control Procedures**

1. Record each morning in the QCPM Book the highest (H) and lowest (L) temperature from the Maximum Minimum thermometer maintained in the refrigerator and the freezer compartments. The procedure for using the Taylor Maximum-Minimum thermometer is as follows:
   a. To record the minimum index (L), refer to the left hand side of the thermometer. *Read the bottom edge of the index.*
   b. To record the maximum index (H), refer to the right hand side of the thermometer. *Read the bottom edge of the index.*
   c. Record the minimum index in the QCPM Book under "Low," and the maximum index under "High." Initial all entries.
   The upper left hand side of the thermometer is in minus degrees. The upper right hand side of the thermometer is in positive degrees.
2. After taking the two readings, reset each index by placing the ceramic magnet across the U-tube in a horizontal position and draw downward slowly, until the indices come to rest on the tops of the mercury columns.
3. If mercury becomes separated, grasp the thermometer firmly at the upper end giving a number of forceful downward swings, until the columns are reunited.

**Person(s) Responsible**

Medical technologist or collector to be designated by the supervisor.

**Preventive Maintenance**

Keep thermometers clean and handle with care. Turn in any broken thermometers to the Safety Coordinator.

*(From Hermann Hospital Clinical Laboratories, with permission.)*

one type of instrument that must be maintained by blood collection personnel. The sphygmomanometer is another instrument used in blood collection procedures that must be maintained and checked for quality assurance. Table 9-7 shows an accuracy check for a sphygmomanometer that should be used by a phlebotomist if he/she uses one during blood collection procedures.

Another instrument frequently used and maintained by phlebotomists is the centrifuge. The centrifuge that is used to spin down the blood must be checked for accurate speed in addition to the preventive maintenance procedures. The speed of the centrifuge can be checked by a tachometer which indicates the speed in revolutions per minute (RPM). The relative centrifugal force or "g" value is then determined from a nomogram as shown in Figure 9-2. The g value gives the efficiency of the instrument by determining the true force exerted by the centrifuge.[2]

## SAFETY IN SPECIMEN COLLECTION

The goal of safety in the health-care institution is to recognize and eliminate hazards and provide information on safety education so that employees can have a healthy work environment. The responsibility for safe working conditions must be assured by the employer and has been mandated by law under the Occupational Safety and Health Act (OSHA) of 1970.[3] Knowledge of OSHA requirements and cooperation between the employer and employee concerning these requirements are necessary in health-care facilities to achieve a safe working place. Thus, the phlebotomist needs to become aware of safety policies and procedures in his or her health-care institution.

**TABLE 9-7. ACCURACY CHECKS FOR SPHYGMOMANOMETER**

Sphygmomanometers should be checked quarterly, or more often if handled roughly during transportation or if any defects are suspected.
1. The aneroid gauge is guaranteed to be accurate throughout the scale as long as it is within the "o" reading in the absence of pressure. If ever out of "o," the gauge is returned to the factory for repair and recalibration.
2. The inflating system, exhaust valve, and tubing should be checked for significant leaks in pressure. It should not exceed more than 5 mm Hg per second. Inflate cuff to 250 mm Hg. Hold the pressure for one minute as a test for slow leaks.
3. Test the gauge for accuracy by testing against a "calibrated gauge." Lay the cuff of the "calibrated gauge" flat on a table. Pump air (bulb) into the bag until the dial reads between 40 and 60 mm. Clamp the tube leading to the bulb so that it is air tight. When air is unable to escape, remove the bulb and adapter from the tube and insert another gauge in its place. Unclamp the tube. Both gauges should read the same pressure. The pressure inside the bag is then raised by pressing down on the bag and the increase in pressure should read the same on both gauges. A difference of more than 5 mm Hg in the reading is not acceptable. The gauge in question is returned to the factory for recalibration.

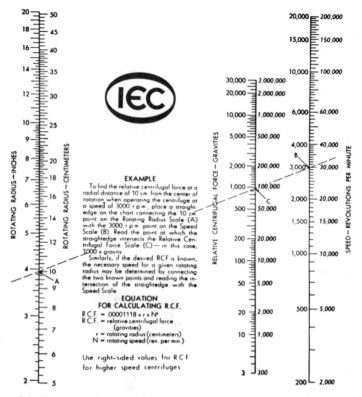

**Figure 9-2.** Nomogram for calculation of relative centrifugal force (RCF) in g. *(From Henry J (ed): Clinical Diagnosis and Management by Laboratory Methods. Philadelphia, Saunders, 1979, p 61, with permission.)*

## Safety in Specimen Handling

Patients' specimens should be handled with precaution to avoid the possibility of acquiring an infection such as hepatitis or those associated with Acquired Immune Deficiency Syndrome (AIDS). For further discussion of precautionary measures for specimen handling, refer back to Chapter 6.

## Personal Hygiene

While on the job, nothing should be inserted into one's mouth (e.g., food, pencils, etc.). Cosmetics should not be applied while on the job. The phlebotomist should avoid biting his or her fingernails or rubbing his/her eyes. Eating, drinking, or smoking within the specimen control section and other laboratory sections must be avoided. No food should be placed in any laboratory refrigerator unless a refrigerator is designated "FOR FOOD ONLY." A laboratory coat should be worn completely buttoned while collecting specimens and removed prior to coffee breaks or lunch. Loose clothing such as scarfs that might become entangled in the centrifuge should never be worn. Long hair must be tied so that it cannot come in contact with specimens or become entangled in the centrifuge. Open-toed shoes are usually prohibited in most clinical laboratories due to the hazards from chemicals and glassware.

## Laboratory Safety

Laboratory safety includes a variety of policies. However, the phlebotomist should remember a few key safety rules at all times. The patients' specimens should be covered at all times during transportation and centrifugation. Centrifuging specimens is best performed within a biohazard safety hood (Fig. 9-3). All waste from specimen collection must be disposed of in the correct containers. One container is usually a heavy double plastic bag that is used for blood specimens disposal, another container for gauze and general trash, and a special container for needles, syringes, and lancets. Urine specimens are usually flushed down the drain with water or flushed down the toilet. Waste should be disposed of gently so that liquids do not splash on other objects. In addition, the work area within the specimen control section should be disinfected periodically according to the clinical laboratory schedule.

If an accident occurs such as sticking oneself with a needle after performing venipuncture on a patient, the phlebotomist should: (a) immediately cleanse area with isopropyl alcohol and apply a Band-Aid and (b) contact the immediate supervisor and the necessary forms should be completed. If an emergency or "STAT" call is made or received, the phlebotomist should not hang up the receiver until all the necessary information has been obtained and the other party has hung up his or her receiver.

## Fire Safety

Fire safety is the responsibility of all employees in the health-care institution. Phlebotomists, therefore, should be familiar with the use and location of fire extinguishers and procedures to follow during a fire. They should be knowledgeable of the exact locations of fire extinguishers and fire blankets. The blankets should be available to smother burning clothes or to use as a fire shield if fire is blocking the exit. Health-care institutions usually have periodic safety education programs in which the phlebotomist can participate and become skillful and knowledgeable in the use of fire safety equipment.

*Fire Extinguishers.* The components of fire are fuel, oxygen, and heat, plus the necessary chain reaction. Four general classifications of fires have been adopted by the National Fire Protection Association.[4] The classifications are:

- *Class A fires,* which occur with ordinary combustible material such as wood, rubbish, and paper;

- *Class B fires,* which occur in a vapor–air mixture over flammable solvents such as gasoline, oil, and paint;
- *Class C fires,* which occur in or near electrical equipment; and
- *Class D fires,* which occur with combustible metals such as magnesium, sodium, and lithium and are infrequently encountered in health-care institutions.

Fire extinguishers correspond with each class of fire.

- *Class A extinguishers.* Soda and acid or water is used to cool the fire.
- *Class B extinguishers.* Foam, dry chemical, or carbon dioxide are used to combat fires composed of vapor–air mixtures over solvents.
- *Class C extinguishers.* Dry chemical or carbon dioxide (nonconducting extinguishing agents) can be used to combat electrical fires.
- *Multipurpose (ABC) extinguishers.* This type of extinguisher is frequently installed in health-care institutions because it reduces the confusion that operation and maintenance of various types entail.

The phlebotomist should learn how to use the various kinds of fire extinguishers in his or her workplace. Use of the wrong type of extinguisher may not only fail to put out the fire but can actually spread it.

Some "do's" and "don'ts" relating to fire safety in health care institutions are:[2]

1. Pull the alarm box located nearest the area you are in.
2. Call the fire number assigned. It should be posted on or near every phone.
3. If the fire is small, attempt to extinguish it, using the proper extinguisher.
4. Should evacuation be necessary, use only stairwells for exiting.
5. Close all doors and windows before leaving the area.
6. If clothing is on fire, drop to the ground and roll, preferably in a fire blanket.
7. If caught in a fire, crawl to the exit. Because smoke rises, breathing is easier at floor level. Breathing through a wet towel is helpful.
8. Do not block entrances, and do not reenter the building.
9. Do not panic.
10. Do not run.

## Electrical Safety

A major hazard in any area of a health-care institution is the possibility of electrical current passing through a person. In the clinical laboratory, the phlebotomist sometimes operates electrical equipment such as a centrifuge. He or she should be aware of the location of the circuit breaker boxes in order to assure a fast response during an electrical fire or electrical shock. The phlebotomist should not use electrical equipment if power cords are

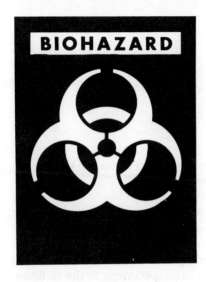

**Figure 9-3.** Sign for biohazardous material.

frayed or if control switches and thermostats are not in good working order.

The centrifuge or other electrical equipment must be unplugged before maintenance is performed. An electrical instrument that has had liquid spilled on or in it and has come in contact with the wiring should be immediately unplugged and dried out prior to any further use.

If an electrical accident occurs involving electrical shock to some employee or patient, the phlebotomist should be aware of the following:

1. The electrical power source must be shut off. If this is impossible, carefully remove the electrical contact from the victim using something such as asbestos gloves that does not conduct electricity or place one's hand in a glass beaker and push the power supply away from the victim. The rescuer should not attempt to touch the victim without the above precautions!
2. Medical assistance should then be called and cardiopulmonary resuscitation (CPR) started immediately. The victim should not be moved prior to medical assistance. A fire blanket or other warm clothing should be put over the victim to keep him or her warm until medical help arrives.

## Radiation Safety

The three cardinal principles in protecting oneself from radiation exposure are time, shielding, and distance. Radiation exposure is cumulative, and thus, the length of exposure at any one time is one major factor in minimizing the hazard. Areas where radioactive materials are in use and stored must have warning signs (Fig. 9-4) posted on the entrance doors. All

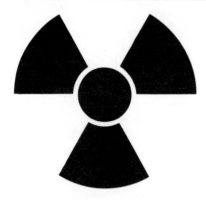

**Figure 9-4.** Signs for possible radiation hazard.

radioactive specimens and reagents must also be properly labeled with the radioactive sign.

Probably, the phlebotomist will encounter possible hazards from radiation exposure only if he or she must collect specimens from patients in the nuclear medicine or x-ray departments, or take specimens to the radioimmunoassay section in chemistry. Thus, the phlebotomist should be cautious in entering an area with the radiation sign and be knowledgeable of the institution's procedures pertaining to radiation safety.

## Mechanical Safety

Because the centrifuge is probably the most frequently used instrument by the phlebotomist, he or she should learn how to maintain this instrument and become familiar with the parts. For example, the phlebotomist should know if the carriers are in the correct position prior to use. If the carriers are not in the correct position, they can swing out of the holding disks into the side of the centrifuge. Also, the wrong head, wrong cups, or imbalanced tubes can lead to the same dangerous problem. If this particular type of accident occurs, patients' specimens or chemicals that are spinning may be propelled onto the side of the centrifuge, broken, and create a dangerous, hazardous problem. Thus, it is of utmost importance to abide by the preventive maintenance schedule and procedures for the centrifuge.

## Chemical Safety

Because the phlebotomist must sometimes pour preservatives such as hydrochloric acid (HCl) into containers for 24-hour urine collections and transport these to the patients' floor, he or she should be knowledgeable of chemical safety.

*Eye Wash and Showers.* The proper clothing must be worn when working with chemicals. A laboratory coat that is buttoned, safety glasses and gloves provide protection and prevent skin contact. When transporting acids or alkalis, an "acid carrier" should be used. It is a specially designed container for carrying large quantities of hazardous solutions.

Safety showers should be near by for use if an accidental chemical spill occurs. Because permanent damage to the skin can result from chemical burns, the victim of a chemical accident must immediately rinse for at least 15 minutes after removing contaminated clothing.

In case of a chemical spill in the eye, the victim should rinse his or her eyes at the eyewash station for a minimum of 15 minutes. Contact lenses must be removed prior to the rinsing in order to thoroughly cleanse the eyes. The victim should not rub the eyes because this may cause further injury. If someone is hurt in a chemical spill, he or she should be taken to the Emergency Department for treatment after rinsing the eyes for 15 minutes.

*Chemical Spill.* If a chemical spill occurs, the phlebotomist should obtain a spill clean up kit from the clinical chemistry section. The kit includes absorbents and neutralizers to clean up acid, alkali, mercury, and other spills. The absorbent and neutralizer used depend upon the type of chemical spill. The absorbent and neutralizer have an indicator system that identifies when the chemical spill has been neutralized and can be considered safe for sweep up and disposal. The phlebotomist should become familiar with the procedures for cleaning up chemical spills in his or her place of employment.

*Disposal of Chemicals.* Chemical waste such as acids and alkalis that are soluble in water can be disposed of by flushing them down the sink with cold water. Acids and alkalis should be poured into a large amount of water before flushing down the sink. The acid *must* be added to water and not vice versa to prevent a violent chemical reaction.

## Disaster Emergency Plan

Many health-care institutions have developed procedures in case of a hurricane, flooding, earthquake, bomb threat, and other disasters. The phlebotomist should become familiar with these procedures because he or she must be prepared for an immediate course of action if conditions warrant it.

## EMERGENCY PROCEDURES

The phlebotomist should become knowledgeable of emergency care procedures because accidents do occur even though precautionary measures are in place. He or she must be able to detach him or herself from the emergency situation to a degree in order to perform well and deliver the best possible health care.

In an emergency situation, the following objectives must be met for the victim: prevent severe bleeding, maintain breathing, prevent shock and further injury, and send for medical assistance.

## Bleeding Aid

Severe bleeding from an open wound can be controlled by applying pressure directly over the wound. A clean handkerchief or other clean cloth (compress) should be placed over the wound before applying pressure by the hand. In an emergency, in the absence of any clean cloth, the bare hand should be used until a cloth compress becomes available. Bleeding of an extremity such as an arm or leg can be decreased by elevation. The injured portion should be raised above the level of the victim's heart unless the injured portion is broken. However, even with elevation, pressure to the wound should be maintained until medical assistance arrives. A tourniquet should not be used to control bleeding except for an amputated, mangled, or crushed arm or leg, or profuse bleeding that cannot be stopped otherwise.

## Breathing Aid

When breathing movements stop or lips, tongue, and fingernails become blue, immediate mouth-to-mouth resuscitation is needed. Delay in using this technique may cost the victim's life. Directions for mouth-to-mouth breathing include the following:

1. See if victim is conscious by tapping on his or her shoulders and yelling "ARE YOU OKAY?" If there is no response, start aid immediately.
2. First step is to place the victim on his or her back and open the airway. Check for obstructions—chewing gum, vomitus, and so on.

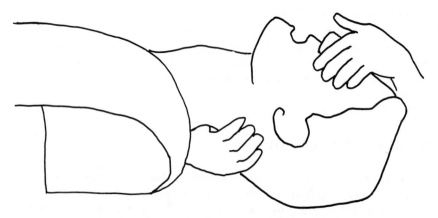

**Figure 9-5.** Head-tilt for emergency care. *(Adapted from the American Heart Association, with permission.)*

3. Put one hand under the victim's neck (Fig. 9-5) and gently lift up. With the other hand placed on the victim's forehead, tilt the head backward to maximum extension. The "head tilt" will clear the airway by moving the tongue away from the back of the throat.

4. Listen and feel for return of air from the victim's mouth and nose for approximately 5 seconds. Also, at the same time, look for the victim's chest to rise and fall.

5. If no breathing, maintain the head tilt, pinch the victim's nose shut with the hand to prevent air from escaping. Open mouth widely, take a deep breath and seal mouth over the victim's mouth (Fig. 9-6). Blow into victim's mouth. Watch for the victim's chest to rise. (If it does not, airway is blocked and must be cleared.)

6. Quickly give four ventilations. If this still does not start an air exchange, reposition the head and try again. After four more ventilations, again look, listen, and feel for breathing. If nothing happens, change the breathing rate to every 5 seconds and continue patiently until the victim starts to breath on his or her own or medical help arrives.

## Circulation Aid

In order to maintain circulation in a victim, the phlebotomist must know the techniques of basic cardiopulmonary resuscitation (CPR). Thus, he or she should check with the supervisor about the availability of CPR classes at the health-care institution because this emergency technique has to be demonstrated to the learner for proper skills to be obtained.

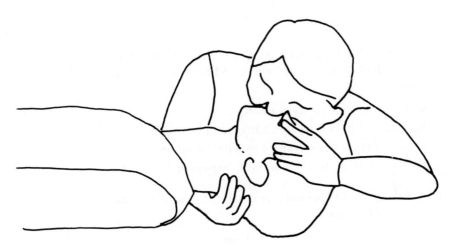

**Figure 9-6.** Breathing aid in emergency situation. *(Adapted from the American Heart Association, with permission.)*

## Preventing Shock

Shock usually accompanies severe injury. It may result from bleeding, extensive burns, insufficient supply of oxygen, and other traumatic events. Early signs include pale, cold and clammy skin, weakness, rapid pulse, increased and shallow breathing rate, and frequently, nausea and vomiting.

The main objectives in treating a shock victim are to improve circulation, provide sufficient oxygen, and maintain normal body temperature.

The following actions are recommended if first aid is given to a shock victim.

1. Correct the cause of shock if possible (e.g., control bleeding).
2. Keep victim lying down.
3. Keep the victim's airway open. If he or she vomits, turn head to the side so that the neck is arched.
4. In the absence of broken bones, elevate the victim's legs so that the head is lower than the trunk of the body.
5. Keep the victim warm.
6. Call for emergency assistance.

Actions that are definitely *NOT* recommended include:

1. Do not give fluids to a victim who has abdominal injury; the person is likely to require surgery or a general anesthetic.
2. Do not give fluids to an unconscious or semi-conscious person.

## STUDY QUESTIONS

The following questions may have one or more answers.

1. A fasting blood specimen for glucose analysis is collected in the morning rather than at a random collection time for which of the following reasons?

   **a.** To avoid the effects of exercise.
   **b.** To avoid the effects of changes in posture.
   **c.** To enhance the effects of diurnal variation.
   **d.** To enhance the phlebotomist's schedule.

2. A fasting blood specimen is needed for which of the following clinical laboratory assays?

   **a.** CBC                    **c.** cholesterol
   **b.** triglyceride           **d.** glucose

3. Which of the following instruments are usually in the specimen control area, and must have preventive maintenance and quality control checks?

   **a.** blood gas analyzer      **c.** centrifuge

   **b.** thermometer      **d.** sphygmomanometer

4. If a fire occurs in or near electrical equipment, which of the following fire extinguishers should be used?

   **a.** class A extinguisher      **c.** class C extinguisher

   **b.** class B extinguisher      **d.** ABC extinguisher

5. What are the major principles in protecting oneself from radiation exposure?

   **a.** distance      **c.** combustibility

   **b.** time      **d.** shielding

## REFERENCES

1. Standard for Evacuated Tubes for Blood Specimen Collection: NCCLS Approved Standards: ASH 1. Villanova, National Committee for Clinical Laboratory Standards, 1980.
2. Lorimor K, Collins F: Monitoring Quality Control in the Clinical Laboratory, in Becan-McBride K: Textbook of Clinical Laboratory Supervision. New York Appleton-Century-Crofts, 1982.
3. Public Law 91-596: Occupational Safety and Health Act. Washington, D.C., U.S. Government Printing Office, 1970.
4. National Fire Protection Association: Hospitals: A fire record. (Reprinted from Fire J.) Boston, National Fire Protection Association, 1970.

# CHAPTER 10

# Management and Education

Doris L. Ross and Amelia T. Carr

The specimen collection or phlebotomy unit provides the interface between the physicians, patients, and nurses and the administration and technical units of the clinical laboratory. Therefore, the management of this unit requires considering the requirements of the people who compose the groups listed, in addition to knowledge and skills related to phlebotomy technique and management expertise. Management or supervision is agreed by most management specialists to consist of planning, organizing, and controlling.[1]

## PLANNING THE OBJECTIVE

In planning a phlebotomy unit, the goals and mission of the hospital, agency, clinic, or company must be considered first. Generally, those goals start with a statement such as "provide efficient and effective patient care" with the understanding that if this goal is met, the corresponding reward of recognition, status, and financial solvency or gain will also be achieved. However, the manager of the phlebotomy unit looks beyond this type of goal or mission to more specific ones that may or may not be recorded as those of the institution. For example, some health-care institutions also have research and educational goals as well as those of patient care. Prior to setting objectives for the phlebotomy unit there are many pieces of information that the manager needs. Most of this information may be obtained by investigating the environment in which the unit operates. The persons who can furnish this information are those who direct the hospital, who own the facility, who direct the patients to the unit (physicians), and/or those who serve the patients (medical technologists, nurses, dieticians, and other health personnel.)

## Planning with Administrators
Administrators may be the source for the following information:

1. the source and number of patients needing the services of the phlebotomy unit (e.g., inpatients, outpatients, patients from health promotional programs in industry, physician-requested analyses on individual patients, or patients in mass screening programs). If the directors or owners do not have this information, it may be necessary to ask physicians, administrators in other settings, directors of the health promotion programs in industry, or directors of the mass screening programs. This type of information is useful in planning for equipment, supplies, and personnel for a phlebotomy team.

2. the age and sex distribution of the bed patients (inpatients) and ambulatory patients (outpatients). The type of phlebotomy equipment and the scheduling may be dictated by the location of the phlebotomy unit (e.g., in a children's hospital, a nursing home, a woman's hospital with primarily obstetrical cases).

3. the socioeconomic, religious, and/or ethnic background of the patients. Special communication skills and/or considerations by the phlebotomist may be necessary for a specific population of patients.

4. the proportion of inpatients to ambulatory patients. This information is useful in planning for personnel and space requirements of the unit. If patients are to come to the phlebotomy unit, consideration should be made on the space and furniture arrangement to accommodate all types of patients, including the physically handicapped.

5. the location of the phlebotomy unit in relation to the laboratory that is to perform the analyses on these specimens. Some phlebotomy units in hospitals are responsible for distributing the specimens to the various laboratories: microbiology, chemistry, serology, hematology, clinical microscopy, blood bank, and/or specialty reference laboratories across the city or out of the city. This information is important in planning transportation time, specimen preservation techniques, the number of personnel needed to transport the specimens to the laboratories, the need for mailing containers, and special mailing or shipping instructions for specimens.

6. the availability of a computer to maintain data files on the patients, their physicians, names and addresses, the date and time of speci-

men collections, and transportation of specimens. Often, in a hospital setting the collecting lists of patients, names of tests, and the patients' room numbers, and specimen labels are generated by a computer. The inventory of supplies, collection schedules, and other administrative uses of the computer add to the efficiency of the phlebotomy unit.

## Planning with Doctors, Nurses, Medical Technologists, Dieticians, and Other Allied Health Professionals

When the phlebotomy unit is placed in a hospital or a matrix environment of other professionals that are performing a service to the same patients and specimens, it is important to learn about their expectations of the phlebotomy unit.

The doctors, nurses, respiratory therapists, radiographers, and physical therapists require time with the patient. It is not uncommon for the phlebotomist to arrive at a patient's room to find that the patient has been transported to the x-ray department or is out of the room for physical therapy. On other occasions, the physician and/or nurse may be changing a dressing or working with the patient in a way that makes it impossible for the phlebotomist to perform his or her job. Identifying a protocol for these situations helps avoid conflict.

Some physicians have certain protocols for their patients. For example, a presurgical protocol may include the following tests: prothrombin time, partial thromboplastin time, blood count, and urinalysis. Another physician may require additional laboratory tests. It is useful to learn from the physicians which types of patients they expect the phlebotomy unit to serve and which kinds of test batteries they usually request. This information provides some indication of the time required to collect the specimens and the kinds of collecting tubes and supplies that are necessary. The medical specialties of the physicians (e.g., pediatrics, oncology, obstetrics, infectious disease, etc.) indicate to some extent the types of supplies that are needed. The planning of a phlebotomy unit is improved if the kinds of specimens can be anticipated.

Medical technologists in clinical laboratories begin to prepare for the analysis of specimens as early as 6:30 or 7:00 AM. They usually expect the phlebotomy specimens to arrive at 8:00 AM or as early as 7:30 AM. It is necessary to coordinate the phlebotomist's schedule with the other health-care responsibilities.

Food service schedules by the dietary service are important to know so that fasting specimens can be collected before the patient's meal tray arrives. A frequent complaint by patients is that their meal trays are delayed or their food becomes cold while they await the phlebotomist.

Coordination of the schedules and expectations of the other health professionals is important to the planning of a phlebotomy unit. After considering the information that can be obtained in advance, the objectives of the phlebotomy unit are outlined and recorded.

Four major objectives of specimen collection identified by Lorimor and Collins are[2]:

1. specimens are collected from the proper patient;
2. specimens are properly identified with the correct information;
3. the necessary specimens are collected in the appropriate containers, in sufficient amounts, and with proper technique; and
4. specimens are available in the laboratory at a time that allows maximum efficiency in determining the result.

An example of the goals of a phlebotomy unit in a large hospital is given in Table 10-1.

## PLANNING FOR STAFF

The staffing of a phlebotomy unit depends upon the factors discussed above. Unless the duties of the phlebotomy section are assumed by evening and night personnel of the clinical laboratory or another unit, staffing for 24 hours is necessary in a hospital setting. Most specimens are collected in the morning, therefore, the largest staff is usually required at that time. However, if a large surgical patient population is served and these patients are admitted for presurgical work-up in the afternoon, the phlebotomy staff would need to accommodate these patients.

In order to maintain a core of staff and also meet increased workloads at these certain hours, some phlebotomy units employ a core of full-time equivalents, FTE, (i.e., full-time employees) and several part-time employees at the peak hours. A method for estimating the number of needed personnel is given later in the discussion of budget preparation.

In many hospitals with large trauma centers or emergency rooms, a

---

**TABLE 10-1. GOALS OF A HOSPITAL PHLEBOTOMY UNIT**

It is the goal of the Department of Laboratory Medicine to establish a service program in support of hospital policy that will enable it to provide experienced technicians in patient care areas to provide the following services:

1. To draw and collect clinical specimens as required by the responsible physicians, in order to facilitate both the diagnoses and treatments of our patients.
2. To provide a liaison service between the responsible physician and the Department of Laboratory Medicine with regard to the scope and level of services available.
3. To deliver specimens to the appropriate laboratory section, and to promptly communicate results of examinations performed.
4. Under the direction of the responsible physician or nurse, to aid in the delivery of patient care as required.

*(Courtesy of L. Jones, B.S., M.T.(AMT) and J. Trujillo, M.D., Director, Department of Laboratory Medicine, The University of Texas System Cancer Center, M.D. Anderson Hospital, Houston, Texas.)*

phlebotomist may be stationed in that area to provide a liaison to the laboratory and to handle the large volume of specimens to be collected there. Phlebotomists may be regularly assigned to a specific patient unit so that the rapport with the patients, nurses, and physicians is strengthened and an effective communication about the laboratory exists.

Thus, phlebotomy staffing requirements depend on:

1. volume of specimens to be drawn;
2. permanent assignment of phlebotomists on daily assignments;
3. the number of times that blood collections are made on any one floor or patient unit;
4. other duties of phlebotomists besides collecting blood, e.g. collecting other specimens from the patient unit (cultures, urines, etc.), discussing specimen collections that require special information, or interpreting the phlebotomy procedure book, or transmittal of specimens from the phlebotomy unit to the laboratories for analyses;
5. the special nature of the patient population (children, burned patients).

The qualifications of the employees of the phlebotomy unit need to be determined. These qualifications are best based on job performance requirements and level of expertise and knowledge required for the service that the phlebotomy unit must provide. The personal qualities expected of a phlebotomist are:

- neat appearance,
- confidence,
- concern for patient,
- courteousness,
- adherence to rules of conduct of the department.

If phlebotomists who have successfully completed a formal phlebotomy training program are employed, the need for long orientation and instruction periods at the beginning of employment is markedly reduced. In addition, trained or experienced phlebotomists have already made a commitment to this work and are not as subject to leave after a few days of employment as are trainees on the job who had little understanding of the work. If non English-speaking patients are anticipated, consideration should be given to at least one employee who can converse in those languages.

## PLANNING FOR SAFETY AND QUALITY

Precautions are necessary in handling specimens to prevent the infection of phlebotomists and transmittal from one patient to another. These precautions are similar to those taken in the areas of the clinical laboratory. They include using acceptable biohazard disposable methods and infection control procedures. These safety precautions are discussed in Chapters 3, 6, and 9.

Quality assurance is indeed a significant aspect of managing a phlebotomy unit. The first three categories in which quality control plays a part in the total quality assurance in the clinical laboratory are (a) patient preparation, (b) specimen collection, and (c) the transportation, handling, and processing of specimens.[2] Discussions of quality control requirements for specimen collection are discussed in Chapter 9.

## PLANNING FOR SPACE AND FACILITIES

The phlebotomy unit should be readily accessible to ambulatory care facilities, elevators, and corridors to inpatient units, and the trauma center. In addition to specimen collection, this division records the requisition, patient data, and information about the patient that are pertinent to the interpretation of test results. Examples of such information are time of last meal, medications, pregnancy, presumptive diagnosis, age, and sex. This concept places the phlebotomy unit as the first data gathering and entry to the information center of the clinical laboratory. Most often this data collection occurs with the use of a computer.

Adequate areas of private cubicles must be provided for the collection of blood from ambulatory patients. These areas are generally furnished with a table on which to keep collecting supplies and a chair with a specially designed arm rest. Cubicles that also accommodate stretchers or wheel chairs should be provided. Some analyses, e.g., serum aldosterone, require that a patient be horizontal and in a quiet area for a period of time prior to blood collection (Fig. 10-1).

There must also be adequate storage space for phlebotomy supplies, including collecting trays. The disposable nature of most of the supplies of the phlebotomy unit requires the availability of a large storage space. There must be collecting trays for each phlebotomist. The phlebotomist's collecting tray becomes personalized by the individual arrangement of supplies, the cleanness, and orderly stocking of supplies. Few phlebotomists elect to share collecting trays.

The supplies are generally ordered a week or two in advance and an inventory of one week's usage is maintained. Because other departments in the hospital may also utilize tubes, needles, and phlebotomy supplies, it is necessary that these stocks be kept secure and inventory records maintained.

Within the phlebotomy or specimen collection unit, the equipment generally required includes refrigerators, centrifuges, sinks, and biohazard disposal waste containers.

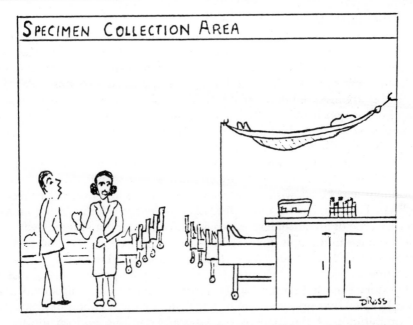

**Figure 10-1.** How could we know this aldosterone specialist was coming to community hospital?

## LEADING, ORGANIZING, BUDGETING, AND MONITORING

### Leading

The manager of the phlebotomy unit should act as a leader. He or she needs to have the phlebotomy skills, the time, and the expertise required to manage effectively. He or she should also be expected to serve as a role model in dealing with patients and other health professionals. The leadership qualities of the manager should be expressed in tact, openness, fairness, and good humor in dealing with all employees. The basic aspects of leadership are:

1. understanding of others,
2. respect for others,
3. knowledge of situations,
4. adaptability,
5. enthusiasm,
6. objectivity,
7. communication skills,
8. confidence in oneself and one's subordinates,
9. proper use of authority, and
10. providing recognition.[4]

Types of leadership styles have been described by McGregor,[5] Blake' and Mouton,[6] and Likert.[7] All have described styles ranging from authoritarian to a more participative management style. The participative type or style of concern for people and production (Blake and Mouton) is generally agreed to be the best leadership approach.[8] In this style, the employees are involved in the planning and organizing of the work. In any case, the manager has the authority and power to assure an acceptable performance by the unit. The judicious and wise use of authority and power are the marks of a good manager.

In managing a phlebotomy unit, it is possible to develop an opportunity for the advancement of those employees who wish to do so. This advancement may be allowing a change of shift hours and assisting in securing financial assistance for employees to enroll in formal academic courses. Another type of advancement is provided by developing several levels for phlebotomists in the unit. For example at The University of Texas System Cancer Center M.D. Anderson Hospital in Houston, Texas, the phlebotomist with experience or 2 years of formal education is classified as an LLT (Laboratory Liaison Technician). This individual enters a program offered in the hospital that prepares him or her to advise nurses and physicians on the preparation of the patients for laboratory testing and on the interference of some procedures with the laboratory analyses. LLTs have access to patients' charts so that specimen collection can be coordinated with the total health care of the patient. This phlebotomist's level has served to improve the quality of care provided to the patient by eliminating multiple venipunctures, repeat collections, and creating an effective working relationship with nurses, physicians, and other allied health professionals.

## Organizing

Some of the aspects of managing discussed in the section on Planning are closely related to organizing. The formal organizational structure is representative of the activities and functions necessary to carry out the objectives and goals of the phlebotomy units.

When the phlebotomy unit is in an institution that also has a clinical laboratory, the phlebotomy unit is customarily a part of the clinical laboratory. A formal organization structure is shown in Figure 10-2. The span of

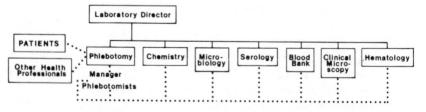

**Figure 10-2.** Organizational chart for phlebotomy matrix.

supervision and the additional position of an assistant manager of the phlebotomy unit depends upon the skill, knowledge, and experience of the employees and the variety of different tasks these people are expected to perform. The most important resource in accomplishing the objectives of the unit are the employees. It is important in the management operation of monitoring to be certain that each employee fully understands what is expected and the criteria that will be used to evaluate his or her performance.

*Schedule of Phlebotomy Collections.* Collections of specimens are usually done at specified times in the hospital. The schedule for the collection of specimens that are to be analyzed that day usually begins with a collection at 7:00 AM followed by others at 11:00 AM, 3:00 PM, and 7:00 PM. The early collection gathers specimens that must be collected while the patient is fasting or before surgery. The others provide collection of specimens ordered by the physician after the early collection or after the patient becomes available for specimen collection, (e.g., returns from physical therapy). Information gathered by a supervisor of a phlebotomy unit for use in planning, staffing, and scheduling is shown in Table 10-2.

Additional or different collection times may be necessary for critical care units. Individual collection trips are made to patients' rooms, surgery, or emergency or trauma room for emergency (STAT) requests.

One of the most difficult problems facing the director and manager of a phlebotomy unit is to achieve a plan to restrict the designation of "STAT" to those truly life-threatening instances. This type of planning requires the most effective communication and cooperation with the hospital administration and medical staff.

## Budgeting

*Types of Budgets.* Zero base budget is one in which all items are justified anew as if no previous budget existed. All items are evaluated and priorities are given. The budget, line by line, is to be justified to the administration. During times of fiscal restraint and possible retrenchment, this type of budget is popular.

Typically, the "forecast budget" has been used in budget preparation. The manager reviews the current budget and adjusts the line item allocations as he or she expects changes to occur over the period of the new budget. The adequacy of the budget prepared in either way is highly dependent upon the information, knowledge, and the synthesis of the information into a scenario involving the phlebotomy unit.

*Direct and Indirect Costs.* Costs considered in the preparation of a budget for a phlebotomy unit include direct costs (e.g., supplies, equipment, etc.)

**TABLE 10-2. AREA HOSPITAL SURVEY OF PHLEBOTOMY MANAGEMENT CHARACTERISTICS**

| Institution | Size (beds) | Technologists Collect | Part-time Employees | Mode of Supervision | Comments |
|---|---|---|---|---|---|
| A. | 270 | 5 PM—6 AM only | No | Supervisor of Specimen Collection unit | 30 daytime technicians, changing shifts and rotations, also staff clinics, do hearing tests, x-rays, and other tests, in addition to blood collection |
| B. | 550 | No | Yes | Technical Laboratory sections responsible for own collection | Strict attendance policy, technicians are given some supervisory experience |
| C. | 1200 | No | No | Supervisor of Specimen Collection unit | Morning collections: 5 AM—7:30 AM, 9 full-time phlebotomists, no regular collections after morning runs |
| D. | 1200 | No | Yes | Supervisor of Specimen Collection unit | 10—11 part-time employees, 10 full-time phlebotomists, absenteeism and tardiness are problems |
| E. | 850 | Yes 2 per floor | No | Supervisor of Specimen Collection unit | Morning collection at 7 AM—8:30 AM, 15 technologists on patient floors. |

*(Courtesy of K. Hlavaty, MT (ASCP), Assistant Supervisor of Hematology, Hermann Hospital, Houston, Texas.)*

and indirect costs. Indirect costs consist of the rental space, laboratory and institutional administrative costs, maintenance and janitorial service, and utilities. These indirect costs are customarily allocated to a department or unit based upon a formula. The formula may use the number of personnel, the square feet serviced, or the number of revenue producing departments to share the allocation.

*Fixed and Variable Costs.* Fixed costs in a budget are those that remain stable over a period of time. These are costs of space, utilities, administration that do not necessarily fluctuate with a change in workload. The variable costs, which include supplies, change in proportion to the volume of work. Fixed costs are larger because almost two-thirds of the fixed costs in a hospital are due to personnel salaries and benefits.

*Revenue.* The cost of collecting specimens usually is not charged as an item to the patient. Generally, it is an addition to the total cost of the analysis to be performed. In some instances when the phlebotomy unit is to collect specimens on animals or engage in some special screening programs, a charge for the collection is made. The revenue for collecting specimens is anticipated and planned in the overall planning of the clinical laboratory or institutional budget.

*Considerations in Budget Preparation.* Customarily, the cost of operating the phlebotomy unit has been allocated among the other accounting centers or units and has not been totally evaluated or financially planned as a separate entity. However, as administrative skills are sharpened and accountability is increased, the identification of costs and the planning of budgets in this operating unit is going to increase in importance.

The items to be considered in the preparation of a budget for phlebotomy are[9]:

1. volume of specimens and other work to be done
2. the human hours required and the skills
3. materials and outside services
4. equipment
5. revenue and rate setting

Once the budget is prepared, it must be presented to the administration for approval and monitored after it is implemented.

## The Workload and Human Hours Required

The volume of specimens that are to be collected per month can be anticipated from the information gained in planning the phlebotomy unit. This figure improves as experience is gained and records are available for identifying trends. Other services that are to be performed are also considered, e.g., mailing, specimens distribution to laboratories for analyses, and record keeping.

Although there are several ways to calculate the human hours required to handle the workload, a weighted time unit, such as the CAP unit, is recommended.[9] Units for laboratory tests including specimen collection are given in the Workload Recording Method for Clinical Laboratories published by the College of American Pathologists (CAP).[10] The CAP unit is described as "one minute of technical, clinical and aide time" for each procedure. The CAP units are given in Table 10.3.

A productivity index may be obtained by the ratio of hours worked per CAP hour. The percentage of productive hours can be calculated by dividing the benefit hours consisting of the vacation hours (120 hr), the sick leave hours (80 hr), and holiday hours (72 hr) by the total hours per year (2050 hr). Using these figures, 13 percent is benefit hours and 87 percent of each paid hour is available for productive work. Now, if a 20-minute break for each 8 hours worked is considered, the figure is lowered to 83 percent or 49.8 minutes of productive time per hour paid.

The CAP also specifies activities that are usually performed in laboratories and that are not related directly to work volume. This time is not counted in the workload. These excluded activities include educational programs, accounting or billing, delivery of reports to physicians or nursing units, research and development, employee scheduling and other administrative duties, purchasing, and computer staff activities.[9]

A typical monthly CAP workload report might show a raw count for specimen collection of 7639, giving CAP workload total units of 62,024. In order to provide 62,024 minutes (1033.7 hours) of work in a 30 day month, 4.3 full-time (40 hr/wk) phlebotomists would be necessary. However, the actual productive time of a full-time employee is only 83 percent. Also, if the specified time not included in the CAP workload count is 10 percent, then the number of productive hours would be 73 percent of the employee's time. Thus, 5.9 persons (full-time equivalents) would be required. Decisions regarding the credentials or level of skills of each of those six persons is then translated into dollar amounts in the budget.

Each person on the payroll is listed with the annual salary for the next fiscal

**TABLE 10-3. CAP WORKLOAD UNITS FOR PHLEBOTOMY**

| Procedure | Units |
|---|---|
| Capillary collection | 12 |
| Venipuncture | 6 |
| Urine collection | 6 |
| Specimen pick-up | 10 |
| Specimen dispatch | 10 |

*(From College of American Pathologists: Laboratory Workload Recording Methods. Skokie, Illinois, College of American Pathologists, 1980, with permission.)*

period. The projected amount of salary increase is added based upon the job performance evaluation.

Depending upon the institution, the employee benefits such as group health insurance and FICA are calculated and placed into the budget by the department or by the institutional fiscal office. These benefits usually are between 15 and 30 percent of the salary. Rates are submitted to the state's rate regulatory agency for approval for reimbursement by health insurers, Medicare, and Medicaid.

Charges for specimen collection vary depending upon the type of collection. An example for the collection of blood for a blood glucose is given in Table 10-4.

The $1.02 figure for the cost of collecting a blood glucose is *only a part* of the total cost involved. It does not include any of the overhead costs for utilities, space, maintenance, and janitorial services. It does not include any administrative, research, or education costs. Estimations of revenue that include the direct and indirect costs are made in collaboration with the departmental and institutional administration. Excellent discussions on budgeting are found in References 9, 11, and 12.

## Monitoring

Monitoring the resources and performance of the phlebotomy unit is a management activity that points to adjustments needed in budgeting, planning, or organizing. It also gives the manager an opportunity to catalog the progress and successes of the unit and its employees.

*Equipment and Supplies.* An inventory of the equipment and supplies in the phlebotomy unit is necessary. A list of each piece of equipment by name, institutional identification tag number, and location should be maintained by the manager and a copy should be given to the laboratory administrator. A review of the accuracy of this list should be made at least annually, with notations and additions made as equipment is discarded, updated, or added. When equipment is discarded or relocated, a record of

TABLE 10-4. DIRECT COST OF COLLECTING A BLOOD GLUCOSE

| | |
|---|---|
| Labor (6 min/collection @ $4.50/hr + $.90 FICA, etc.) | $0.54 |
| Collection tube | 0.17 |
| Needle | 0.15 |
| Alcohol swab | 0.01 |
| Tray ($15.00 depreciated over 5 years) | <0.01 |
| Requisition slip | 0.05 |
| Tourniquet ($0.12 at 800 collections/tourniquet) | 0.01 |
| Gauze squares | 0.04 |
| Bandage, adhesive | 0.04 |
| Total | $1.02 |

this must be kept on file. Records of maintenance service on the equipment are also kept. Maintaining a supply inventory represents a more complex operation. From experience or calculation, volumes of the various kinds of supplies that are needed can be ordered in advance and kept in stock. Space for the storage of supplies is valuable ($5 to $10 per square foot per year)[13] and stocking of large volumes of supplies ties up capital. For these reasons, supplies are generally purchased on a contract basis whereby a designated volume is expected to be purchased over a year's time. The phlebotomy unit requests a certain portion of these supplies to be delivered each week or each month and the institution is billed at that time. Many hospitals maintain approximately two weeks' phlebotomy supplies on hand. A long delivery time on orders increases the stock that must be kept on hand or the timing of the ordering. An excellent discussion of monitoring equipment and supplies may be found in References 12 and 13.

*Monitoring Performance.* The importance of employees and the leadership abilities of the manager have been discussed. The performance of employees is evaluated according to the criteria established by the phlebotomy unit, described in the phlebotomy manual, and provided to the employee at the time of employment.

When situations occur indicating that an employee has failed to meet the criteria, a record should be made and kept in the employee's file. This file should also hold records of performances that were better than average, more than expected, or that showed extra devotion or unique contribution to the job. At regular intervals, the manager meets with the employee and reviews the employee's performance by the established criteria. This meeting should also afford the employee an opportunity to discuss problems or concerns with the manager.

The University of Texas System Cancer Center M.D. Anderson Hospital has a survey form that is given to patients to inquire about the quality of the phlebotomists' services. Most hospitals have an employee that visits patients to assure that the hospital services are acceptable. The phlebotomy manager may receive information in this manner. General areas of concern or reoccurring problems may serve as topics of in-service education or staff meetings.

In-service programs offer phlebotomy employees information on the latest advances in health care that affect their work or enhance their interest in their work. Generally, the employees are asked for topics of interest to them in preparation of the in-service programs. The manager can enhance interest by obtaining interesting guest speakers to present these topics. An evaluation of the in-service programs helps the manager improve the programs. Frequently, there is a coordinator of in-service education for the laboratory or the hospital who can assist in this activity.

Staff meetings are usually held weekly in order to afford communication between employees, the manager, and/or director. The employees should have an opportunity to bring problems or new ideas to the attention of the management. This also provides a time for management to share information about anticipated changes, new rules and regulations, and special events in the laboratory and hospital. Communication with the phlebotomy employees is the manager's most important function.

## PLANNING A FORMAL PHLEBOTOMY EDUCATION PROGRAM

Medical technologists have recognized in recent years that the quality of their laboratory test results, those which provide information for diagnosis and treatment of patients, is directly affected by the quality of the collected blood sample. Many medical technologists expressing this concern to their respective administrations have met with approval and support in developing a formal training program for phlebotomists in the individual institution or as a service to the area's medical community.

### Steps For Achieving Support From Management
Several steps should be followed to facilitate the development of a phlebotomy program. The *first step* is to develop a statement of need and the identification of goals. A few suggested methods for acquiring verification of a suspected need are:

1. Circulate a questionnaire pertinent to specimen collection to laboratory department personnel and nursing staff for a hospital situation. A university department interested in developing a training program can circulate a similar questionnaire to hospitals or other clinical facilities in the surrounding area.
2. Interdepartmental meetings or representatives concerned with specimen collection problem-solving can produce minutes suggesting formal phlebotomy education.
3. Documented incidents or problems directly related to the current level of phlebotomy education can be reviewed.

After the statement of need has been adequately supported with documentation, identification of the goal(s) is in order. The goal(s) should be fashioned to fulfill the statement of need while ultimately assuring quality laboratory blood specimen collection and thereby quality health care to the patient.

The *second step* to achieve support is to review the verification of need and submit a preliminary proposal for a formal educational program to the administration. If the response is favorable, continue with the development of the proposal.

The *third step* is the identification of educational resources. In a hospital-based program, the educational or in-service department personnel may be requested to advise and assist in writing objectives, providing classrooms, and suggesting a format for a course syllabus. It would be advisable to have input and thereby commitment from personnel in the other hospital departments who would be working with the phlebotomy students (e.g., Nursing). In a university-based program, the medical technology faculty are accustomed to writing objectives, outlines, and formats. The majority of the work in this situation would involve juggling classroom time schedules and achieving affiliation agreements with clinical facilities for phlebotomy student clinical rotations.

The *fourth step* requires a literature review of standards and guidelines for phlebotomy instruction as well as a review of other types of phlebotomy education programs.[14-16] The National Committee for Clinical Laboratory Standards (NCCLS) standard procedures for the collection of diagnostic blood specimens by venipuncture provides guidelines for proposing and conducting a phlebotomy training program as well as criteria for interviewing and selecting candidates.[14] Clinical Laboratory Sciences Career Entry *Statements of Competence*[17] and *Body of Knowledge Content Outline*[18] also provide guidelines from a professional organization.

The *fifth step* begins the development of a course syllabus. A syllabus should contain the following information:

1. Prerequisites/Requirements (minimum acceptable)
2. Intended audience (intra-institution or public offer)
3. Class schedule (dates course is offered as well as agenda of a single course offering)
4. Purpose of course
5. Course objectives
6. Instructor/Faculty/Institution/Affiliation information
7. Course fee (if public offering)
8. Course description, content outline, and student policies
9. Credits/Units/Certificates
10. Contact for further information or application.

The *sixth and final step* in proposing a formal phlebotomy educational program involves finances. At this point, hours of instruction and staffing costs must be calculated. Costs of purchasing equipment and supplies needed in a fiscal year per student take on new importance. Income resulting from tuition fees must be included in the financial evaluation. A realistic viewpoint is necessary to decide what facets of the educational program will fit budgetary allowances and still provide quality phlebotomists.

## Providing the Basic Education and Training Program

The phlebotomy student must understand the objectives to be met and the expectations of the instructors at the beginning of the course. These objectives should be identified both verbally and in writing. The NCCLS Standards for objectives of a training program require that upon completion of training the student should be able to:

1. explain the physical layout of a blood drawing area and/or hospital floors;
2. identify equipment used in collection of blood and describe its use;
3. identify the various documentation forms associated with blood collection;
4. identify collection sites normally used in blood collection;
5. perform collection techniques on a simulated arm to include all basic steps in venipuncture and skin puncture.

## Student Policies

Student policies may be written to express the objectives, goals, and expectations of the student.[19] In this way, policy reinforces the path to meeting the objective and attaining the goals. Policies should cover:

1. personal qualifications,
2. dress code,
3. time and attendance,
4. replacement of supplies and documents,
5. examinations and references for exam questions,
6. student liability,
7. health care of the student during the training session.

A special area in the policies should spell-out grounds for failure. Time and attendance should explain a mechanism for excused and unexcused absence consequences. Makeup time and examination procedures should be covered carefully. Interjecting time and attendance policies provides a process for screening out the irresponsible phlebotomist who would not exercise responsibility in a patient care situation.

## Teaching Facilities

If the phlebotomy education process takes place in only one institution, arrangements need to be made for classroom space, for didactic instruction, and access to patients for clinical instruction.[20] Phlebotomy educational situations that include more than one facility may require an affiliation agreement, the input and support of supervisory personnel, and consideration of a variety of time schedules in the teaching agenda.

## Equipment and Instructional Materials

Equipment and instructional materials important to a phlebotomy education experience include all the items that are listed for a venipuncture procedure or a skin puncture procedure (Fig. 10-3). (See Chapter 3). Additional items that would be desirable for proper training are:

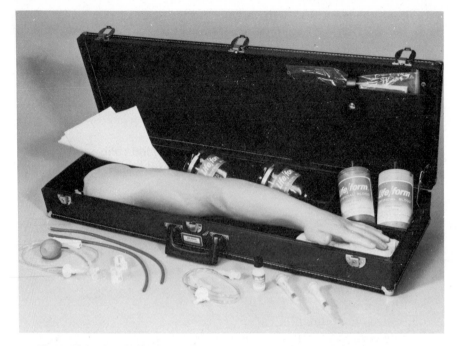

**Figure 10-3.** Nasco Life/form injectable training arm. A phlebotomy student needs to learn collection techniques using proper training equipment prior to patient collection. *(Courtesy of Nasco, Inc.)*

- Nasco Life/form training arms (adult and pediatric arms with human colored skin). (Refer to Fig. 10-3.)
- Collection trays
- Anatomical models
- Anatomical and circulatory charts
- Projectors—slide and film
- Chalkboards and/or tablets and markers
- Teaching manuals and references

All of the equipment, supplies, and instructional materials must be planned and ordered well in advance of the time needed for instruction and must be stored when not in use.

## Communication and Advertising

It is important to have a continuous flow of communication between the coordinator and the other instructors and affiliations. The nursing staff of the clinical facility should be informed in advance in order to render them cooperative with a program developed to improve patient care. Advertising the phlebotomy education program is a necessary activity if the program is to be marketed to clinical facilities or the public or both. This requires planning and publishing brochures detailing the course syllabus, as well as contacting the media and planning elements of exposure to the audience.

## Selecting the Students

Selecting the students for each class requires specific selection criteria and a team of representatives involved in the selection. The criteria for most phlebotomy training programs require a high school diploma or General Education Development (GED) test certificate. The personal characteristics that are covered in the student policies may also be employed in the selection criteria.

A personal interview with the candidate for selection is important to a successful phlebotomy program. The NCCLS approved standard: ASH-3 Standard Procedures for the Collection of Diagnostic Blood Specimens by Venipuncture Appendix A1—Training program states that a candidate for a phlebotomy training program when interviewed should be poised, alert, pleasant, mature, enthusiastic, and sincere. Questioning the candidate should bring to surface characteristics of initiative, ability to speak well, cooperative attitude, and attention to detail. Because professional appearance is important for an occupational phlebotomist, a personal interview provides an opportunity to screen applicants in the areas of appearance and hygiene. An interview with a candidate also allows an opportunity for questioning the candidate and evaluating the responses. An acceptable candidate demonstrates good communication skills and self-confidence. Prior clinical experience and favorable references should be the first areas questioned. The desire to learn the skill of phlebotomy as a possible stepping stone into other medical careers is commonly expressed by candidates. Locomotion and agility must be considered because a phlebotomist walks and stands an excessive amount of time in most working situations. Strength (ability to lift up to 60 pounds) is often necessary for lifting equipment, supplies, and some patients. Reading, spelling, color-blindness, and mathematics entrance exams may be desirable because documentation, basic calculations, and differentiating tube colors in collection are essential capabilities for the practicing phlebotomist. A typical position summary or job description for a phlebotomist is as follows: collects and handles specimens, consults with supervisor and related health-care team members, and maintains supplies needed for blood collection. Keeping a summary such as this in mind, it is easy to see why the above criteria must be specific. Also, as in other health-care careers, phlebotomy candidates must be willing to work different shifts and weekends if necessary.

## Phlebotomy Program Content

It is suggested that a phlebotomy training program consist of both didactic and clinical instruction. The phlebotomy student should receive didactic instruction encompassing the topics covered in Chapters 1 through 9 prior to patient contact in the clinical instruction.

In the clinical setting, the phlebotomy student will have an opportunity to develop confidence through experience. The student should be carefully supervised in the initial attempts to collect blood specimens from patients. These first patients should be carefully selected for their large veins and cooperative attitudes. The supervising professional should remain close enough during these first experiences to take over as needed. Instruction on this level should contain elements of positive reinforcement, confidence in ability, reassurance and the ever important respect for self-esteem. The phlebotomy student needs much encouragement in the initial exposure to the patient.

Areas of information pertinent to the particular clinical facility that should be emphasized to a phlebotomy student during clinical instruction are:

1. Tasks on a checklist listing expected rate and level of performance of the student
2. Laboratory and institutional policies
3. Job description for phlebotomist
4. Medicolegal aspects relative to the particular institution
5. Safety, fire, and disaster plans: the role of the student in the event of an incident
6. First aid
7. Infection control and reporting
8. Specimen Collection Manual or File and standard protocol
9. Procedures for documentation: requisitions, logs, etc.
10. Professional conduct and appearance.

*Class Schedule.* The length of the course in hours needs to be determined as soon as the program content has been developed. The times, dates, and locations of the individual classes must be carefully worked through. Phlebotomy educational programs mentioned in the literature review range from 40 hours to 150 hours in duration. Most programs have divided the time in the class schedule into periods half of which are didactic instruction and the other half, clinical instruction. Some programs offer full day instruction, whereas others offer instruction for only 4 hours each day.

The National Phlebotomy Association (NPA) requires that a phlebotomy education program have a minimum of 48 hours of didactic instruction and at least 100 hours of clinical instruction to be eligible for accreditation. Graduates of NPA-accredited programs are eligible for the NPA certification exam.[21]

The daily agenda should spell-out reading assignments as well as activities for each day. This agenda, as part of the syllabus, aids the student in preparing for class as well as simplifies the task of course revision. Instructors can "fill-in" for each other as needed if the lecture and laboratory outlines are available and the agenda is specific.

*Certificates/Credits/Units.* A graduation ceremony for presentation of phlebotomy course certificates is highly recommended. The ceremony instills pride in the graduate and allows an opportunity to invite interested representatives from future clinical affiliates. The certificate should contain the following:

1. Name of the course and the institution(s) (should include clinical affiliate).
2. Seals from the institution(s).
3. Number of hours of instruction/credits/units. (There are mechanisms for achieving college credits or continuing education units for a phlebotomy course from either a university, professional organization, or other educational accrediting group. Course credit is based upon contact hours of instruction.)[22]
4. Full name of the graduate.
5. Date of graduation.
6. Appropriate signatures, (e.g., administrator, dean, director, instructor).

A phlebotomist graduating from a certificate program will be able to take this certificate to a prospective employer. With the advent of formal phlebotomy education programs, a phlebotomist now has a need for credentials when seeking employment.

*Teaching Methods.* It is recommended that for each skill taught, there should be five basic phases to the teaching process utilized in a phlebotomy education program.

| Phase | Competency Tested |
|---|---|
| 1. Preparation | Oral quiz, homework questions, written quiz. |
| 2. Familiarization | After seeing instructor demonstrations, oral quiz, homework questions, and written quiz. |
| 3. Observation | Oral quiz, student teaching instructor approach. |
| 4. Manipulation | Role-playing and practical exams for student to demonstrate technical competence. |
| 5. Operation | Clinically supervised bedside instruction according to checklist of tasks to master techniques in clinical setting.[23] |

The student must progress from one phase to another only after demonstrating competency. This is described as competency-based education. In the case of inability to demonstrate competence within the framework of the course, the student may be given another chance to achieve and demonstrate competence. He or she should be aware that the score of a second evaluation must be averaged with the initial attempt and in that case only a previously set passing score may be achieved. Should the student fail to demonstrate the required level of competency on a second chance, the student should not continue in the program. Only students who have been able to demonstrate competence within the guidelines of the program for a particular phase of instruction are eligible to progress to the next phase. All areas of information should be covered in a comprehensive final examination. Failure to demonstrate competency on the final examination should preclude graduation from the program.

Several methods of instruction are recommended for use in a phlebotomy education program. Included are: lecture, group discussion, demonstration, role-playing, case studies, independent study, and self-examination. Instructional aids include slide – tape programs, videocassettes, transparencies, and opaque projections, films, models, and various charts and drawings.

## Evaluation Techniques

*Evaluating the Student.* Phlebotomy students must be able to demonstrate skills in all three behavioral domains: cognitive, affective, and psychomotor. In the cognitive domain, the student must demonstrate knowledge, theory, understanding, and problem-solving skills; all of which can be evaluated through written exam or practical demonstration. However, evaluation of this nature cannot impose the stress, tension, and multitude of other variables affecting the performance of a phlebotomist in a "real life" situation. This is why evaluation of the affective domain is important to phlebotomy education.[24] Behavior reflecting attitude, coping capabilities, and methods of adjustment and adaptation must be tested and evaluated. Only the phlebotomist who is capable of maintaining an optimum attitude and necessary composure can successfully perform phlebotomy skills and manipulations. Role-playing between students and instructors is a good predecessor to patient contact and a way to give preliminary feedback about the student's attitude. A phlebotomist who has role-playing experience as a student often finds it easier to go step by step through a procedure in the real life situation (Fig. 10-4).

Much of the behavior demonstrated in the affective domain is dependent upon personality. The important attitudinal characteristics should be listed in the screening process of phlebotomy applicants, if possible. Evaluating these characteristics is a difficult task that may be accomplished by

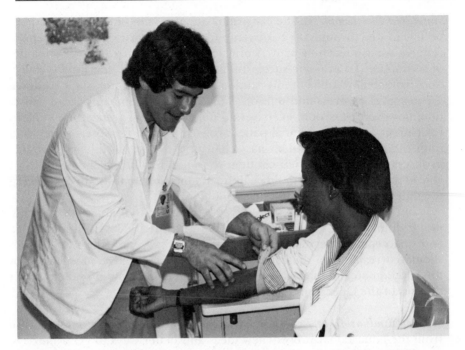

**Figure 10-4.** Role-playing exercises aid the student in learning patient approach skills.

using behavioral objectives incorporated in the policies and procedures taught. In this way, infractions which break policy will demonstrate incompetency. For example:

> Upon completion of the phlebotomy training program, the student will be expected to perform venipuncture procedures in accordance with the NCCLS Standard Procedures for the Collection of Diagnostic Blood Specimens by Venipuncture while exhibiting good communication skills, personable attitude, ethical conduct, self-confidence, organization, and responsibility, as well as professional appearance and hygiene.

A policy written in a similar fashion to the above (shorter versions are certainly advisable) would incorporate both performance and behavioral objectives. Behavioral objectives may be written to require a professional behavior and appearance of a phlebotomy student which can then be used as an evaluation tool for the affective domain in phlebotomy education.

Phlebotomy manipulative skills are evaluated in the psychomotor domain. This area may be tested with simulated practicum in the classroom and with performance checklists in the clinical setting.[25]

*Simulated Practicum.* In the classroom situation, the phlebotomist should be able to step through the basic venipuncture and basic skin puncture procedures using a teaching arm. A practicum of this nature allows evaluation of technique. To evaluate successful collection of blood specimens, collection from fellow phlebotomy students tests psychomotor skills under a greater level of stress and tension. This exercise resembles patient collection, however, classroom exercises do not completely prepare the student for patient contact and initial patient collection must be closely supervised until the phlebotomy student has achieved a level of confidence that aids in successful collection. Self-confidence is vital for the phlebotomist to be able to perform. There should be defined limits in the program concerning the time when this self-confidence should evolve.

In the clinical rotation, a tool frequently used to evaluate the psychomotor domain is a task list of procedures with specific levels of acceptable and unacceptable performance per task. The tasks and the rating levels should correspond to the course and procedure objectives. Evaluation of the psychomotor domain during the clinical rotation should take place at the end of the Operation Phase of instruction.

*Student Evaluation of Program.* Phlebotomy students sometimes surmise from the educational process new ideas and better ways to get a message across. They are also good at pinpointing trouble spots in the instruction of the program.

Many times the good students are complimentary and constructive, while the poor students are disgruntled and critical. However, an instructor can find useful information from an evaluation of a program by the students. After the comprehensive final exam but before the final grades have been posted is a good time to request filling out an evaluation of the program. Student evaluations of a program can be used in improving it as well as justifying it as a service to the institution and community.

*Instructor Evaluation of the Program.* Input and evaluation of the program by its instructors is invited. However, providing an evaluation tool that lists questions with ratings and a place for comments stimulates the instructors to respond or take the time to note an idea for improvement. Instructor evaluations are also valuable to justify a program, especially if the evaluations come from instructors in affiliated clinical institutions. Remember, it is important to involve the instructors in the evaluation and revision of the phlebotomy education program to ensure their continued commitment to its success.

## Seeking Employment
Interviewing skills and resume writing may be covered in the program to prepare phlebotomy students to embark on a new career. Role-playing

helps here too. It is frustrating to a phlebotomist graduating at the top of the class to be passed up for a position because he or she lacks interviewing skills or experience composing a resume.

## CONTINUING EDUCATION

The phlebotomist graduating from a formal training program needs to realize the importance of remaining current in the field. Continued education is directly related to continued competence.[26] Keeping the occupational phlebotomist updated is critical to competency in phlebotomy practice which changes and improves constantly since it is an area of the medical field.

Workshops that teach trouble-shooting in phlebotomy are valuable to the practicing phlebotomist.[27] Communication skills are so important that revitalizing patient approach skills especially with different kinds of patients is good preventive maintenance for the phlebotomist. Because the phlebotomist is the most visible member of the laboratory, not just to the patients but to other health-care team members, in-service involving improving interdepartmental relationships should include the phlebotomist.

Phlebotomy is a stressful position as described in Chapter 8. Patient contact and the pressing importance of proper specimen collection render stress management exercises helpful to phlebotomists. Such exercises may aid a phlebotomist in communicating more effectively and discharging phlebotomy duties in a pleasant manner.

## STUDY QUESTIONS

1. List 6 factors to be considered in planning a phlebotomy unit.
2. List 4 goals of a typical phlebotomy unit.
3. List 5 factors that dictate staffing requirements.
4. The phlebotomy collection procedure manual is used for [choose correct answer(s)]:

   a. recording the approved procedures for the phlebotomy unit.

   b. readily accessible performance by phlebotomists.

   c. criteria for acceptable performance by phlebotomists.

   d. a handy pocket reference to be carried by the phlebotomist.

5. List 10 basic characteristics of leadership.
6. List 4 factors that affect the scheduling of collections.
7. List 5 items to be considered in the preparation of a budget.

8. Given a raw count of 3800 capillary collections, 5000 venous punctures, 100 specimen pick-ups, 50 specimen dispatches, and 50 urine collections, over an 8-hour shift in a 30-day month, how many full-time equivalents of personnel will be needed?
9. What is the direct cost of collecting a capillary blood glucose?
10. Name 3 reasons for monitoring.

*For the remaining questions, circle the single best answer.*

11. The statement of need for a phlebotomy education program expresses concern for the

    a. number of blood samples requiring collection.

    b. the variety of specimen collection criteria.

    c. affect of blood collection on test results.

    d. amount of time taken to correct phlebotomy errors.

12. The ultimate goal of a phlebotomy education program is to increase

    a. the number of phlebotomists.

    b. the time a medical technologist is at the bench.

    c. quality health care to the patient.

    d. the standards for phlebotomists.

13. The NCCLS standards for a phlebotomy training program are found in the NCCLS Approved Standard for Standard Procedures for

    a. skin puncture.

    b. venipuncture.

    c. collection devices.

    d. phlebotomy training programs.

14. The content outline for the didactic portion of the course should vary from the clinical rotation in order to emphasize

    a. clinical laboratory and institutional policies.

    b. interdepartmental relationships.

    c. equipment and supplies to use.

    d. application of acquired knowledge.

15. An example of proper training equipment for teaching venipuncture technique is a(an)

    a. model of the circulatory system.

    b. injectable arm.

    c. venipuncture demonstration film.

    d. ample supply of syringes and Vacutainer systems.

**16.** Instructional materials can be used to

a. enhance understanding prior to application.

b. replace clinical application.

c. explain the process after application.

d. determine the ability to apply knowledge.

**17.** Methods of instruction used may be

a. lecture and group discussion.

b. demonstration and role-playing.

c. case studies and independent study.

d. all of the above.

**18.** The recommended phase training theory utilizes 5 phases:

(1) Familiarization      (4) Manipulation

(2) Preparation      (5) Observation

(3) Operation

These phases must progress in which order:

a. (2), (5), (4), (3), (1)

b. (2), (4), (5), (3), (1)

c. (2), (4), (3), (5), (1)

d. (2), (4), (5), (1), (3)

**19.** Selection criteria for phlebotomy education program candidates must include

a. minimum acceptable prerequisites.

b. locomotion capabilities.

c. minimum length of hair.

d. a and b only.

**20.** The interview is important in selecting phlebotomy candidates mainly because it allows the interviewer(s) to evaluate

a. communication skills

b. prior knowledge of phlebotomy.

c. ethical conduct.

d. student's finances.

## REFERENCES

1. Becan-McBride K (ed): Textbook of Clinical Laboratory Supervision. New York, Appleton-Century-Crofts, 1982, p 9.
2. Lorimor KK, Collins FL: Monitoring quality control in the clinical laboratory, in Becan-McBride K (ed): Textbook of Clinical Laboratory Supervision. New York, Appleton-Century-Crofts, 1982, pp 146–244.
3. Reece RL: The screening laboratory of 1980. Perspect Biol Med 17:227, 1974.

4. Martin BG, Karni K: Leadership, in Karni KR, Viskochil KR, Amos PA (ed): Clinical Laboratory Management. Boston, Little, Brown, 1982, p 287.
5. McGregor D: The Human Side of Enterprise. New York, McGraw-Hill, 1960.
6. Blake R, Mouton J: The Managerial Grid. Houston, Gulf, 1964.
7. Likert R: New Patterns of Management. New York, McGraw-Hill, 1961.
8. Murphy MB: Personnel relationships, in Becan-McBride (ed): Textbook of Clinical Laboratory Supervision. New York, Appleton-Century-Crofts, 1982, pp 107–113.
9. Duplantis D: Budgetary considerations, in Becan-McBride K (ed): Textbook of Clinical Laboratory Supervision. New York, Appleton-Century-Crofts, 1982, p 238.
10. College of American Pathologists: Laboratory Workload Recording Methods. Skokie, IL, College of American Pathologists, 1980.
11. Anderson F: Budgets, in Karni KR, Viskochil KR, Amos PA (eds): Clinical Laboratory Management. Boston, Little, Brown, 1982, pp 393–399.
12. Reich MD, McLendon WW: Fiscal management, in Henry JB (ed): Clinical Diagnosis and Management by Laboratory Methods. Philadelphia, J.B. Saunders, 16th ed, 1979, pp 1995–2006.
13. Loder RJ: Purchasing and inventory control, in Karni KR, Viskochil KR, Amos PA (eds): Clinical Laboratory Management. Boston, Little, Brown, 1982, pp 393–399.
14. National Committee for Clinical Laboratory Standards, NCCLS Approved Standard: ASH-3 Standard Procedures for the Collection of Diagnostic Blood Specimens by Venipuncture, Appendix A1—Training Program, March 1980.
15. Valaske MJ: So You're Going to Collect a Blood Specimen. College of American Pathologists, January 1982.
16. Donald MK, Adkins D, Smith JP: Development of a curriculum for the preparation of phlebotomists. AJMT 48:11, November 1982.
17. Career Statements of Competence: Clinical Laboratory Sciences. Bellaire, Texas, ASMT, 1978.
18. Body of Knowledge Content Outline: Clinical Laboratory Sciences. Houston, Texas, ASMT, 1980.
19. Phlebotomy Training Sessions: University of Texas School of Allied Health Sciences Program in Medical Technology, P.O. Box 20708, Houston, Texas 77225, 1982–1983.
20. Phlebotomy Section Training Program: Forrest General Hospital Clinical Laboratory, P.O. Drawer 1897, Hattiesburg, Mississippi 39401, 1979.
21. The National Phlebotomy Association (N.P.A.): Continuing Education Programs. N.P.A., 7610 Georgia Avenue, N.W. Suite 2, Washington, D.C. 20012, 1980.
22. Golden TH: A college course for phlebotomists. MLO 1981.
23. Grimaldi PQ: Phase training: A systematic approach to lab instruction. MLO 1981.
24. Bobek JR: Evaluating behavioral traits in students, AJMT 38:11, November 1972.
25. Synder JR Wilson JC: Evaluation of student performance in the clinical setting using the process skills approach. J Allied Health 1980.
26. Petition Submitted to the 1981 House of Delegates: ASMT for the Formation of a Phlebotomist Section of the Scientific Assembly.
27. Larson JM: A stick in time saves nine. MLO 1981.

# APPENDIX 1

# Basic Requests in English, Spanish, French, and Vietnamese

Diana Garza

The following phrases are designed to present the phlebotomist with a *VERY BASIC* means of communicating with Spanish-, French-, and Vietnamese-speaking patients. Before speaking with patients, it is recommended that the phlebotomist practice using these phrases with someone who knows the correct pronunciation. Otherwise, the patient may be even more confused.

| English | Spanish | French | Vietnamese |
|---|---|---|---|
| Good day/morning | Buenos dias | Bonjour | chao buôi sang |
| Good afternoon/evening | Buenas tardes/noches | Bonsoir | chao buôi tôi |
| Man, Mr., Sir | Señor | Monsieur | ông |
| Girl, Miss, Ms. | Señorita | Mademoiselle | Cô |
| Lady, Mrs., Madame | Senora | Madame | Ba |
| My name is . . . | Me llamo . . . | Je m'appelle . . . | Tôi tên la . . . |
| I work in the laboratory. | Trabajo en el laboratorio. | Je travaille au laboratoire. | Tôi lam viêc tai phong thi nghiêm. |
| What is your name? | Como se llama? | Comment vous appelez-vous? or (Quel est votre nom?) | Tên (ông, Ba, Cô) la gi? |
| I need to: | Necesito: | Il faut que: | Tôi cân lây môt mâu mâu se cân dâm |
| . . . take a blood sample | . . . sacar sangre | . . . je prenne du sang | vao dâu ngon tay |
| . . . stick your finger | . . . picarle su dedo | . . . je prenne du sang de votre doigt | |
| We are going to analyze: | Vamos analizar: | Nous allons analyser: | Chung tôi se phân chât: |
| . . . your blood | . . . su sangre | . . . votre sang | . . . Mau cua (ông, Ba, Cô) |
| . . . your urine | . . . su orina | . . . votre urine | . . . Nuoc tiêu cua (ông, Ba, Cô) |
| . . . your sputum | . . . su esputo | . . . votre crachat | . . . Dom cua (ông, Ba, Cô) |

| | | | |
|---|---|---|---|
| Please: | Favor de: | . . . s'il vous plait | Xin naim bun tay lai |
| Make a fist (close your fist) | Cerrar el puño | Faites le poing | Xin naim bun tay lai |
| Bend your arm | Doblar el brazo | Pliez le bras | Xin co canh tay lai |
| Roll up your sleeve | Levantarse la manga | Roulez la manche | Xin xan tay ao lêu |
| Open your hand | Abrir la mano | Ouvrez la main | Xin mo bau tay ra |
| Go to the bathroom | Ir al baño | Allez à la salle de bain | Hay di vao phong tain |
| Urinate in this receptacle | Orinar en este recipiente | Urinez dans ce recipient | Xin tiêu vao cai by nay |
| Sit down here | Sientese aqui | Asseyez-vous ici | Xin ngôi xuông dây |
| Change your position | Cambiarse de posicion | Changez votre position | Hay dôi chô |
| Turn over | Voltearse | Tournez vous | Xin nam xoay lai |
| Change to the left | Cambiarse a la izquierda | Tournez à gauche | Xin quay rê bên trai |
| Change to the right | Cambiarse a la derecha | Tournez à droit | Xin quay rê bên phai |
| The doctor wrote the order. | El doctor escribio la orden. | Le docteur a ecrit l'ordre. | Bac si da viêt don nay. |
| | La doctora " " | La doctoresse " " | |
| Have you had breakfast? | ¿Ya tomo el desayuno? | Avez-vous manger le petit dejeuner? | (ông, Ba, Cô) da au sang chua. |
| You should not eat. | No debe de comer. | Ne mangez rien avant la prise de sang. | (ông, Ba, Cô) khong nêu au thue au. |
| | | OR Il ne faut rien manger. | |
| It hurts a little. | Duele un poquito. | ÇCa fait un peu mal. | |

# APPENDIX 2

# Units of Measurement

## Diana Garza

| | |
|---|---|
| amp | ampere (units of electric current) |
| °C | degrees Centigrade or Celsius (unit of temperature; convert to Fahrenheit by multiplying by 1.8 and adding 32) |
| c | centi- ($10^{-2}$) |
| cc | Cubic centimeter (same as ml, 1/1000 liter) |
| cd | candela (units of luminous intensity) |
| cm | centimeter |
| cu mm or mm³ | cubic millimeter |
| d | deci- ($10^{-1}$) |
| da | deca- ($10^{1}$) |
| dl | deciliter (1/10 of a liter) |
| °F | degrees Fahrenheit (unit of temperature; convert to Centigrade by subtracting 32 and multiplying by 0.555) |
| g or gm | gram (1/1000 of a kilogram, unit of mass) |
| hpf | high power field on microscope |
| G% | grams in 100 ml |
| h | hecto- ($10^{2}$) |
| IU | international unit |
| k | kilo- ($10^{3}$) |
| °K | degrees Kelvin (thermodynamic temperature; convert to Centigrade by subtracting 273.15) |

| | |
|---|---|
| kg | kilogram (1000 grams, or 2.2 pounds) |
| L | liter (1000 ml or 1000 cc, unit of volume) |
| lpf | low power field on microscope |
| m | meter (unit of length) |
| m | milli- ($10^{-3}$) |
| $\mu$ | micro- ($10^{-6}$); micron |
| $\mu$g or mcg | microgram (1/1000 milligram) |
| mCi | millicurie |
| mEq or meq | milliequivalent |
| mg or mgm | milligram (1/1000 gram) |
| mg% | milligrams in 100 ml (same as dl) |
| min | minutes |
| mIU | milliinternational unit (1/1000 IU) |
| ml | milliliter (1/1000 liter, same as cc) |
| mm | millimeter (1/10 centimeter) |
| cu mm or mm$^3$ | cubic millimeter |
| mm Hg | millimeters of mercury |
| mmole | millimole |
| mol, M | mole (units of substance) |
| mOsm | milliosmol |
| N | normality |
| n | nano- ($10^{-9}$) |
| ng | nanogram (1/1000 microgram) |
| p | pico- ($10^{-12}$) |
| pg | picogram (1/1000 nanogram) |
| QNS | quantity not sufficient |
| sec | second (unit of time) |
| SI | international system |
| sp g | specific gravity |
| u | international enzyme unit |
| $\mu$ | micro |
| $\mu$g (mcg) | microgram (1/1000 milligram) |
| wt | weight |
| w/v | weight/volume |
| $\mu$Ci | microcurie (1/1000 of a millicurie) |
| WNL | within normal limits |
| WNR | within normal range |
| $\leqslant$ | less than or equal to |
| $\geqslant$ | greater than or equal to |

# APPENDIX 3

# Metric Conversion Chart

Diana Garza

| | |
|---|---|
| Length | 1 inch (in) = 2.54 centimeters (cm) |
| | 1 foot (ft) = 30.48 centimeters (cm) |
| | 39.37 inches (in) = 1 meter (m) |
| | 1 mile (mi) = 1.61 kilometers (km) |
| Mass | 1 ounce (oz) = 28.35 grams (g) |
| | 1 pound (lb) = 453.6 grams (g) |
| | 2.205 pounds (lb) = 1 kilogram (kg) |
| Volume | 1 fluid ounce (fl oz) = 29.57 milliliters (ml) |
| | 1.057 quarts (qt) = 1 liter (liter or L) |
| | 1 gallon (gal) = 3.78 liters (liter or L) |

# APPENDIX 4

# Formulas and Calculations

## Diana Garza

| | |
|---|---|
| Area | square meter (sq m or $m^2$) |
| Clearance | liter/second (L/s) |
| Concentration and Conversions | |
|    Mass | kilogram/liter (kg/L) |
|    Substrate | mole/liter (mol/L) |

$\%^{w/v}$ to M or vice versa:

$$M = \frac{\%^{w/v} \times 10}{\text{molecular wt.}}$$

$\%^{w/v}$ to N or vice versa:

$$N = \frac{\%^{w/v} \times 10}{\text{eq. wt.}}$$

mg/dl to mEq/L or vice versa:

$$mEq/L = \frac{mg/dl \times 10}{\text{eq. wt.}}$$

M to N:

$$N = M \times \text{Valence}$$

N to M:

$$M = \frac{N}{\text{Valence}}$$

| | |
|---|---|
| Density | kilogram/liter kg/L |
| Dilutions | Final concentration = Original concentration × Dilution 1 × Dilution 2, etc. |

| Electrical potential | Volt | $V = kg\ m^2/s^3 A$ |
| Energy | Joule | $J = kg\ m^2/s^2$ |
| Force | Newton | $N = kg\ m^2/s^2$ |
| Frequency | Hertz | $Hz = 1\ cycle/s$ |

Hematology Math

Mean corpuscular volume ($\mu m^3$):

$$MCV = \frac{Hct \times 10}{RBC\ in\ millions}$$

Mean corpuscular hemoglobin (pg):

$$MCH = \frac{Hemoglobin\ (g) \times 10}{RBC\ in\ millions}$$

Mean corpuscular hemoglobin concentration (%)

$$MCHC = \frac{hemoglobin\ (g) \times 100}{Hct}$$

Pressure    Pascal    $Pa = (kg/m)s^2$

Quality Control Math

Variance ($s^2$)

$$s^2 = \frac{(x - \bar{x})^2}{n - 1}$$

Standard deviation(s)

$$s = \sqrt{s^2}$$

% Coefficient of variation

$$\%CV = \frac{s}{\bar{x}} \times 100$$

Solutions

Percent (%)

To find amount of solute needed to make a given volume of solution:

$$g\ (or\ ml)\ of\ solute\ to\ be\ diluted\ up\ to\ desired\ volume = \frac{\% \times desired\ volume}{100}$$

To find % solution when amount of solute and total volume of solution are known:

$$\% = \frac{g\ (or\ ml)\ solute \times 100}{volume}$$

Molarity (M)

$$g/L = molecular\ weight \times M$$

$$M = \frac{g/L}{molecular\ wt.}$$

$$mmole/L = \frac{mg/L}{molecular\ wt.}$$

Osmolarity (Osm/L)

$$Osm/L = M \times particles/molecule\ after\ ionization$$

$$mOsm/L = mmole/L \times particles/molecule\ after\ ionization$$

$$Osm/L = \frac{\Delta\ temperature}{1.86}$$

$$mOsm/L = \frac{\Delta\ temperature}{0.00186}$$

Normality (N)

$$eq.\ wt. \times N = g/L$$

$$N = \frac{g/L}{eq.\ wt.}$$

Specific gravity (sp $g$)

$$sp\ g = \frac{wt.\ of\ solid\ or\ liquid}{wt.\ of\ equal\ volume\ of\ H_2O\ at\ 4°C}$$

**Temperature**

Celsius or Centigrade

$$(°C = °K - 273.15; °C = °F - 32 \times 0.555)$$

Kelvin

$$°K = °C + 273.15\ or\ 5/9\ °F + 255.35$$

Fahrenheit

$$°F = [°C \times 1.8] + 32$$

**Volume**

cubic meter cu mm or $m^3$

liter $\quad L = dm^3$

# APPENDIX 5

# Abbreviations and Medical Terminology

Diana Garza

| | |
|---|---|
| a | Without (e.g., aphasia, inability to speak) |
| ∝ | Alpha |
| ab- | Deviating (e.g., abnormal) |
| ABG | Arterial blood gases |
| ABO | Blood types |
| ABR | Absolute bed rest |
| a.c. | Ante cibum, L., Before meals |
| AC | Alternating current |
| ACD | Acid citrate dextrose, anticoagulant |
| ACTH | Adrenocorticotrophic hormone |
| ACU | Acupuncture |
| ad- | Toward (e.g., adduction) |
| aden/o- | Gland (e.g., adenopathy) |
| ADH | Antidiuretic hormone |
| ad lib | At pleasure; as described |
| ADP | Adenosine 5-diphosphate |
| aer/o | Air (e.g., aerobic) |
| AFB | Acid-fast bacillus |
| AFP | Alpha-fetoprotein |
| Ag | Silver |
| A/G | Albumin/globulin ratio |
| Agg | Agglutination |
| AGL | Acute granulocytic leukemia |

| | |
|---|---|
| AHG | Antihemophilia globulin |
| AIDS | Acquired immune deficiency syndrome |
| AIHA | Autoimmune hemolytic anemia |
| AK | Above the knee |
| Al | Aluminum |
| al- | Pertaining to (suffix; e.g., hormonal) |
| ALA | delta-aminolevulinic acid |
| ALL | Acute lymphocytic leukemia |
| ALT | Alanine amino transferase (term for SGPT) |
| alges- | Overly sensitive to pain (e.g., algesia) |
| algia- | Pain (suffix; e.g., neuralgia) |
| AM | Morning |
| AML | Acute myeloblastic leukemia |
| an- | Without (e.g., anemia) |
| ANA | Antinuclear antibodies |
| angi/o- | Vessel |
| ante- | Before (e.g., anterior) |
| anti- | Against (e.g., antisepsis) |
| Approx | Approximately |
| APPT | Activated partial thromboplastin time (PTT) |
| ARD | Antibiotic removal device |
| arthro- | Pertaining to joint(s) (e.g., arthritis) |
| As | Arsenic |
| ASAP | As soon as possible |
| ASO | Antistreptolysin O titer |
| AST | Asparate amino transferase (term for SGOT) |
| ATP | Adenosine triphosphate |
| Au | Gold |
| aur- | Ear |
| Auto-Trans | Autologous transfusion |
| AV | Atrioventricular, arteriovenous |
| B | Boron |
| Ba | Barium |
| baso- | Basophils |
| $\beta$ | Beta |
| BBT | Basal body temperature |
| B cell | Lymphocyte derived in bone marrow |
| BC | Blood culture |
| BCP | Biochemical profile; and birth control pills |
| BFP | Biologically false positive |
| Bi | Bismuth |
| bi- | Two (e.g., bifurcate) |
| b.i.d. | Bis in die; twice daily |
| bio- | Life (e.g., biology) |

| | |
|---|---|
| BM | Bowel movement |
| BMR | Basal metabolic rate |
| bp | Boiling point |
| B/P | Blood pressure |
| Br | Bromide |
| brady- | Slow (e.g., bradycardia) |
| bronch- | Windpipe (e.g., bronchitis) |
| BS | Blood sugar |
| BSA | Body surface area |
| BSP | Bromsulphalein dye for liver function |
| BUN | Blood urea nitrogen |
| C | Carbon, compliance, clearance, Coulomb |
| c̄ | With |
| Ca | Calcium, cancer |
| CAB | Coronary artery bypass |
| carcin/o- | Cancer (e.g., adenocarcinoma) |
| caudal | Near tail |
| $C_3$ $C_4$ | Complement factors |
| C&S | Culture and sensitivity |
| cardio- | Heart (e.g., cardiopulmonary) |
| CAT | Computerized axial tomography scan |
| CBC | Complete blood count |
| CCU | Coronary care unit |
| CDC | Center for Disease Control |
| CEA | Carcinoembryonic antigen |
| cele | Herniation (suffix; e.g., meningiomyelocele) |
| centesis | Surgical puncture (suffix; e.g., amniocentesis) |
| cephalo- | Head (e.g., cephalic) |
| cerebro- | Cerebrum, brain (e.g., cerebrospinal fluid) |
| CEU | Continuing education units |
| CF | Complement fixation |
| $CH_3OH$ | Methanol |
| $(C_2H_5)OH$ | Ethanol |
| $C_6H_{12}O$ | Glucose |
| CIE | Counter immunoelectrophoresis |
| Cl | Chloride |
| CML | Chronic myelogenous leukemia |
| Co | Cobalt |
| co- | Together, with (e.g., coagulation) |
| $CO_2$ | Carbon dioxide ($PCO_2$ = partial pressure of $CO_2$) |
| $CO(NH_2)_2$ | Urea |
| contra- | Against (e.g., contraceptive) |
| CNS | Central nervous system |
| CPD | Citrate phosphate dextrose, anticoagulant |

| CPK | Creatine phosphokinase |
| CPR | Cardiopulmonary resuscitation |
| Cr | Chromium |
| cranial | Near head |
| crin/o | Secrete (suffix; e.g., endocrine) |
| CRP | C-reactive protein |
| Crit | Hematocrit |
| CSF | Cerebrospinal fluid |
| Cu | Copper |
| CV | Curriculum vitae, L, biographical data |
| cyan/o- | Blueness (e.g., cyanotic) |
| cyst/o- | Fluid sac, bladder (e.g., encystment) |
| cyt/o- | Cells (e.g., cytopathology) |
| δ | Delta |
| D&C | Dilatation and curettage |
| DC | Direct Current |
| derm/o- | Skin (e.g., dermatophyte) |
| dia- | Through (e.g., diaphragm) |
| DIC | Disseminated intravascular coagulation |
| Diff | Differential (white blood cells) |
| Dis | Disease |
| Distal | Away from body trunk |
| DNA | Deoxyribonucleic acid |
| DOA | Dead on arrival |
| dorsal | Back |
| DPT | Diphtheria, pertussis, tetanus vaccine |
| DRG | Diagnosis related groups |
| dyn/o | Pain (e.g., carotodynia) |
| dys- | Painful, difficult (e.g., dysmenorrhea) |
| EBV | Epstein-Barr virus |
| ECG, EKG | Electrocardiogram |
| ECHO | Echocardiogram |
| ectasia- | Dilatation (suffix) |
| ect/o- | Outside (e.g., ectoparasite) |
| EDTA | Ethylenediaminetetraacetate |
| EEG | Electroencephalogram |
| ELISA | Enzyme-linked immunosorbent assay |
| EM | Electron microscopy |
| em- | In (e.g., empyema) |
| emia | Blood (suffix; e.g., leukemia) |
| end/o- | Inner (e.g., endotrachial tube) |
| ENT | Ear, nose, throat |
| entero/o | Small intestine (e.g., enteritis) |
| eos | Eosinophils |

| epi- | Over, near, upon (e.g., epidemic) |
| ER | Emergency Room |
| erythro- | Red (e.g., erythrocyte) |
| ESR | Erythrocyte sedimentation rate |
| ex/o- | Out from |
| extra- | Outside, beyond (e.g., extrasensory) |
| F | Fluorine |
| FA | Fluorescent antibody test |
| FBS | Fasting blood sugar |
| Fe | Iron |
| FEP | Free erythrocyte porphyrins |
| FLK | Funny looking kid |
| FSH | Follicle stimulating hormone |
| FSP | Fibrinogen split products |
| FTA | Fluorescent treponemal antibody |
| FUO | Fever of unknown origin |
| $\gamma$ | Gamma |
| gastr/o- | Stomach (e.g., gastroenteritis) |
| GC | Gonococcus (gonorrhea) |
| geri- | Old age (e.g., geriatrics) |
| gest- | Bear, carry, (e.g., gestation) |
| GFR | Glomerular filtration rate |
| GFT | Graft (e.g., skin) |
| GH | Growth hormone |
| GI | Gastrointestinal |
| glyco- | Sweet, sugar (e.g., glycolysis) |
| G-6-PD | Glucose-6-phosphatase dehydrogenase |
| GTT | Glucose tolerance test |
| gtts | Drops |
| GVH | Graft versus host reaction |
| gynec/o- | Woman (e.g., gynecology) |
| H | Hydrogen |
| HAA | Hepatitis-associated antigen |
| HAT | Heterophile antibody titer |
| $H_3BO_3$ | Boric acid |
| Hb (Hgb) | Hemoglobin |
| HBD | Hydroxybutyric dehydrogenase |
| $HB_sAg$ | Hepatitis B surface antigen |
| HCG | Human chorionic gonadotropin |
| HCl | Hydrochloric acid |
| Hct | Hematocrit |
| HDN | Hemolytic disease of the newborn |
| He | Helium |
| H&E | Hematoxylin and eosin stain |

| | |
|---|---|
| hema- | Blood (e.g., hematology) |
| hemi- | Half (e.g., hemisphere) |
| hepato- | Liver (e.g., hepatocyte) |
| Hg | Mercury |
| 5HIAA | 5-hydroxyindoleacetic acid |
| $HNO_3$ | Nitric acid |
| $H_2O$ | Water |
| hr | Hours |
| h.s. | At bedtime |
| $H_2SO_4$ | Sulfuric acid |
| hydro- | Watery (e.g., hydrocephalic) |
| hyper- | Above, more than normal (e.g., hyperplasia) |
| hypo- | Under, less than normal (e.g., hyponatremia) |
| I | Iodine |
| ia | Condition (suffix; e.g., leukemia) |
| iasis | Formation or presence of (suffix; e.g., psoriasis) |
| IBC | Iron binding capacity |
| ICSH | Interstitial cell-stimulating hormone (LH in females) |
| ICU | Intensive care unit |
| Ident | Identification (ID) |
| IFA | Immunofluorescence antibody test |
| Ig | Immunoglobulin (e.g., IgA, IgM) |
| inferior | Away from head |
| inter- | Between (e.g., interdependent) |
| intra- | Within (e.g., intrauterine) |
| I&O | Intake and output |
| ist | One who (suffix; e.g., microbiologist) |
| itis | Inflammation (suffix; e.g., conjunctivitis) |
| IV | Intravenous |
| IU | International unit |
| IUD | Intrauterine device |
| $\kappa$ | Kappa |
| K | Potassium |
| 17-KGS | 17-ketogenic steroids |
| ly-KS | 17-ketosteroids |
| LAL | Limulus amoebocyte lysate test |
| later- | Side, away from body midline (e.g., lateral) |
| lb | Pounds |
| $\lambda$ | Lambda |
| LDH, LD | Lactic dehydrogenase |
| LDL | Low-density lipoprotein |
| LE prep | Lupus erythematous test |
| leuk- | White (e.g., leukocytosis) |
| LFT | Liver function tests |

| | |
|---|---|
| LH | Luteinizing hormone (ICSH in males) |
| Li | Lithium |
| lipo- | Fatty (e.g., lipoproteins) |
| lith- | Stone, calculus (e.g., lithiasis) |
| LP | Lumbar puncture |
| lymph- | Lymph (e.g., lymphocyte) |
| lysis | Breaking down (suffix; e.g., hemolysis) |
| Lytes | Electrolytes (Na, Cl, K, bicarbonate) |
| MBC | Minimal bactericidal concentration |
| macro- | Large (e.g., macrocyte) |
| mal- | Bad, abnormal (e.g., malaria) |
| malac/o | Softening, (e.g., malacoma) |
| mast/o- | Breast (e.g., mastectomy) |
| MCH | Mean corpuscular hemoglobin (RBC indices) |
| MCHC | Mean corpuscular hemoglobin concentration (RBC indices) |
| MCV | Mean corpuscular volume (RBC indices) |
| medial | Toward body midline |
| megal/o | Enlarged (e.g., megaloblastic) |
| mening/o- | Membrane (e.g., meningitis) |
| metr- | Uterus (e.g., endometrium) |
| metr/o- | Measure (e.g., metric) |
| Mg | Magnesium |
| MHA | Microhemagglutination test |
| MI | Myocardial infarction |
| MIC | Minimal inhibitory concentration |
| MIF | Migration inhibition factor |
| micro- | Small (e.g., microcytic) |
| MMR | Measles, mumps, rubella vaccine |
| mono | Monocytes |
| mo | Months |
| Mr. | Mister |
| Ms. | Mrs/Miss |
| multi- | Many |
| myc/o- | Fungal (e.g., mycosis) |
| myelo- | Marrow (e.g., myeloblastic) |
| myo- | Muscle (e.g., myocardium) |
| N | Nitrogen |
| NA | Not applicable |
| Na | Sodium |
| NaCl | Sodium chloride (salt) |
| $NaHCO_3$ | Sodium bicarbonate |
| NaOH | Sodium hydroxide |
| nat- | Birth (e.g., natal) |

| | |
|---|---|
| NC | Normal color |
| Neg | Negative |
| ne/o- | New (e.g., neoplasm) |
| nephr- | Kidney |
| neuro- | Nerve |
| NG | Nasogastric |
| $NH_3$ | Ammonia |
| Ni | Nickel |
| NL | Normal, normal limits |
| NMR | Nuclear magnetic resonance |
| no | Number |
| noso- | Disease (e.g., nosocomial) |
| NPN | Nonprotein nitrogen |
| NPO | Nothing per os (mouth) |
| NR | Nonreactive |
| $O_2$ | Oxygen ($PO_2$ = partial pressure) |
| OB | Obstetrics |
| 17-OH | 17-hydroxysteroids |
| oid | Like, resembling (suffix; e.g., Lymphoid tissue) |
| ologist | One who studies (suffix; e.g., microbiologist) |
| ology | The study of (suffix; e.g., microbiology) |
| oma | Tumor related (suffix; e.g., lymphoma) |
| onco- | Tumor related (e.g., oncology) |
| O&P | Ova and parasites |
| ophthalm/o | Eye (e.g., ophthalmology) |
| OR | Operating room |
| orrhagia | Hemorrhage (suffix) |
| os | Mouth |
| osis | Condition, usually abnormal (suffix; e.g., dermatosis) |
| oste/o- | Bone (e.g., osteomyelitis) |
| ostomy | Surgical forming of an opening (suffix; e.g., colostomy) |
| OTC | Over-the-counter (drugs) |
| otomy | Surgical forming of an opening (suffix; e.g., colostomy) |
| P | Phosphorus |
| PA | Pernicious anemia |
| pan- | all; complete (e.g., pandemic) |
| para- | Beside, around, near (e.g., paracystitis) |
| paralysis | Loss of movement |
| path/o- | Disease (e.g., pathology) |
| path/o- | To bear; to carry (e.g., pathogen) |
| Pb | Lead |
| PBI | Protein-bound iodine (outdated) |
| p.c. | After meals |
| PCV | Packed cell volume (hematocrit) |

| | |
|---|---|
| pedi/a- | Child (e.g., pediatrics) |
| ped/o- | Foot (e.g., pedicle) |
| penia | Decrease in (suffix; e.g., leukopenia) |
| peri- | Around (e.g., periorbital) |
| pH | Hydrogen ion concentration |
| phleb/o- | Vein (e.g., phlebotomy) |
| PID | Pelvic inflammatory disease |
| PKU | Phenylketonuria |
| plas/o- | Formation (suffix; e.g., neoplasty) |
| plast/o- | Surgical repair, reconstruction (suffix; e.g., mammoplasty) |
| Pl.ct. | Platelet count |
| Plts. | Platelets |
| PM | Evening |
| PMNs | Polymorphonuclear cells (type of WBC) |
| pneumo- | Lungs, air (e.g., pneumonia) |
| pod/o- | Foot (e.g., podiatry) |
| poly- | Too many (e.g., polyploid) |
| Pos | Positive |
| post- | Behind; after (e.g., posterior) |
| PP or PC | Postprandial (or after meals) |
| PPLO | Pleuropneumonia-like organism (characteristics between virus and bacteria) |
| pre- | Before; in front of (e.g., prenatal) |
| PRN | As needed |
| pro- | In front of (e.g., proenzyme) |
| proct- | Rectum, anus (e.g., proctoscope) |
| proximal | Near body truck |
| pseudo- | False (e.g., pseudopregnancy) |
| PSI | Pounds per square inch |
| PSP | Phenolsulfonphthalein (dye for renal excretion test) |
| psych/o- | Soul; mind (e.g., psychology) |
| PT | Prothrombin time |
| PTH | Parathyroid hormone or parathormone |
| ptosis | Prolapse; sagging (suffix; e.g., ophthalmoptosis) |
| PTT | Partial thromboplastin time (see also APTT) |
| py/o- | Pus (e.g., pyogenic) |
| pyr/o- | Fire; fever (e.g., pyrophobia) |
| q.d. | Quaque die, every day |
| q.h. | Quaque, hora, every hour |
| q.2h. | Every 2 hours |
| q.i.d. | Quater in die, four times daily |
| QNS | Quantity not sufficient |
| q.o.d. | Every other day |

| | |
|---|---|
| quad | Quadruple |
| R | Reactive |
| RA | Rheumatoid arthritis |
| Radi- | Ray (e.g., radiotherapy) |
| RAI | Radioactive iodine |
| RAST | Radioallergosorbent test |
| RBC | red blood cell |
| re- | Back; again (e.g., remission) |
| ren/o- | Kidney (e.g., renal) |
| Retic | Reticulocyte count |
| retr/o- | Behind; in back of (e.g., retroperitoneal) |
| RF | Rheumatoid factor (also called RA factor) |
| Rh | Rhesus; Rh factor in blood |
| RIA | Radioimmunoassay |
| RNA | Ribonucleic acid |
| R/O | Rule out |
| RPR | Rapid plasma reagin (test for syphilis) |
| RT | Room temperature |
| Rx | Medication |
| S | Sulfur |
| Σ | Sigma, sum of |
| s̄ | Without |
| S&A | Sugar and acetone |
| sagittal | Lengthwise |
| scler/o- | Hard (e.g., sclerosis) |
| scop/o- | To examine; look at (suffix; e.g., proctoscopy) |
| sed/rate | Sedimentation rate |
| segs | Segmented neutrophils of WBC |
| semi | Half (e.g., semisynthetic) |
| sep- | Decay (e.g., septic) |
| SG | Specific gravity |
| SGOT | Serum glutamic-oxaloacetic transaminase (newer name is AST) |
| SGPT | Serum glutamic-pyruvic transaminase (newer name is ALT) |
| SI | System of International Units |
| Si | Silicon |
| SIDS | Sudden infant death syndrome |
| sine | Without |
| SMA | Sequential multiple analyzer (SMA-6 does 6 tests, SMA-12, 12 tests) |
| SOB | Shortness of breath |
| spasm | Contraction; twitching |
| SS | Social Security |

| | |
|---|---|
| stasis | Stopping; controlling (suffix; e.g., hemostasis) |
| Stat | Immediately, now |
| sten/o- | Narrow (e.g., stenosis) |
| STS | Serologic test for syphilis |
| sub- | Below; under (e.g., suborbital) |
| super- | Above; more than normal (e.g., superior) |
| supra- | Above; more than normal (e.g., suprapubic) |
| Surg | Surgery |
| $T_3$ | Triiodothyronine |
| $T_4$ | Thyroxine |
| tact | Touch (e.g., tactile) |
| tach/y- | Rapid; fast (e.g., tachycardia) |
| TAT | Tattoo |
| TB | Tuberculosis |
| TBG | Thyroid-binding globulin |
| TBI | Total body irradiation |
| T&C | Type and cross-match |
| T cell | Lymphocyte derived from thymus |
| thromb/o- | Clot (e.g., thrombosis) |
| TIBC | Total iron-binding capacity |
| t.i.d. | Ter in die, three times daily |
| tox- | Poison (e.g., toxicology) |
| TP | Total protein |
| TPI | Treponema pallidum immobilization |
| TPR | Temperature, pulse, respiratory |
| trans- | Across (e.g., transtracheal) |
| TRH | Thyroid-releasing hormone |
| tri- | Three (e.g., trisomy) |
| troph/o- | Nourishment; development (e.g., trophology) |
| T&S | Type and screen |
| TSH | Thyroid-stimulating hormone (thyrotropin) |
| TSP | Total serum proteins |
| TSS | Toxic shock syndrome |
| UA | Urinalysis |
| UC | Urine culture |
| uni- | One; single (e.g., unilocular) |
| UrAc | Uric acid |
| URI | Upper respiratory infection |
| ur/o- | Urine (e.g., urology) |
| UTI | Urinary tract infection |
| UV | Ultraviolet |
| vas/o- | Vessel (e.g., vasoconstriction) |
| VD | Venereal disease |
| VDRL | Venereal Disease Research Laboratory (test for syphilis) |

| | |
|---|---|
| ven/o- | Vein (e.g., venipuncture) |
| ventral | Front |
| viscer- | Viscera |
| VLDL | Very low-density lipoprotein |
| VMA | Vanillylmandelic acid |
| WBC | White blood cell; white blood count |
| WNL | Within normal limits |
| WNR | Within normal range |
| X match | Cross-match (of blood) |
| X | Female chromosome |
| Y | Male chromosome |
| yr | Years |
| Zn | Zinc |

# Appendix References

Abbott Laboratories: Common Medical Terminology and Abbreviations. North Chicago, IL. 60064, 1982.

Campbell JB: Laboratory Mathematics, Medical and Biological Applications. 2nd ed, St. Louis, C.V. Mosby, 1980.

Corbett JB: Laboratory Tests in Nursing Practice. Norwalk, CT, Appleton-Century-Crofts, 1982.

Frenay AC: Understanding Medical Terminology. 6th ed, St. Louis, Catholic Health Association of the U.S., 1977.

Henry JB: Todd-Sanford-Davidsohn Clinical Diagnosis and Management by Laboratory Methods. 16th ed, Philadelphia, W.B. Saunders, 1979.

Kaplan A, Szabo LL: Clinical Chemistry Interpretations and Techniques. Philadelphia, Lea & Febiger, 1979.

Remson ST, Ackermann PG: Calculations for the Medical Laboratory. Boston, Little, Brown, 1977.

Tietz NW: Fundamentals of Clinical Chemistry. Philadelphia, W.B. Saunders, 1976.

# Answers to Study Questions

**CHAPTER 1**
1. a
2. b
3. c
4. a
5. b

**CHAPTER 2**
1. a, b
2. d
3. a, d
4. b, d
5. c

**CHAPTER 3**
1. a, b, c
2. d
3. b
4. c
5. b
6. a
7. b
8. c

**CHAPTER 4**
1. a, b
2. b, c
3. a, b, c
4. b, c
5. d
6. a
7. d
8. a, c, d
9. b, d
10. a, b, c, d

## CHAPTER 5

1. The thumb has a pulse that may be confused with the patient's own pulse.
2. Once the site is decided upon, the area should be cleaned well with Betadine and allowed to dry.
3. The Duke method is difficult to standardize and does not allow ample surface area to repeat the test, if needed. If bleeding is excessive, it is difficult to control at this site.
   The Ivy method provides ample testing area on the volar surface of the forearm. The length and depth of incision can be standardized with a commercial template. Excessive bleeding can be readily controlled at this site.
4. After locating a vein, the phlebotomist should release the tourniquet and scrub the entire area well with soap for about 2 minutes. A sterile alcohol pad is used to remove the soap from the puncture site moving out in increasing circles. The alcohol is allowed to dry and Betadine is applied in the same manner and allowed to dry.
5. Skin tests are a simple, relatively inexpensive way to determine if a patient has ever had contact with particular antigens and has produced antibodies to that antigen.
6. The patient should be instructed to eat normal, well-balanced meals for 3 days prior to the test. Eight hours before the test is to start, the patient should be fasting completely except for water. Water intake is encouraged throughout the test. No other beverage is allowed. Cigarette smoking and gum chewing should be discouraged until the completion of the test.
7. Because both tolerance tests rely on the injection of the stimulants into a vein, the phlebotomist may only assist the physician or other qualified personnel in the test and draw the required blood specimens as directed.
8. In the diagnosis of cystic fibrosis.
9. a. Weight—donors should weigh at least 110 lb.
   b. Temperature—oral temperature may not exceed 37.5°C.
   c. Pulse—should be strong, regular beats; 50 to 100 beats/minute.
   d. Blood pressure—the systolic blood pressure should be between 90 and 180 mm Hg and the diastolic blood pressure should be between 50 and 100 mm Hg.
   e. Skin lesions—both arms should be examined for signs of drug addiction.
   f. General appearance—if the donor looks ill, excessively nervous, or under the influence of alcohol or drugs, he or she should be deferred.
   g. Hematocrit or hemoglobin—the hematocrit must be no less than 38 percent for females and no less than 41 percent for males. The

hemoglobin value may be no less than 12.5 g/dl for female donors and no less than 13.5 g/dl for male donors.
10. About 405 to 495 ml.
11. Therapeutic phlebotomy is used in the treatment of some myeloproliferative diseases such as polycythemia or other conditions in which the removal of blood benefits the patient.
12. Timed specimens, fasting specimens, stat specimens.
13. Coagulation tubes should be filled first and mixed, then blood should be delivered to other anticoagulated tubes and mixed. Finally, blood is delivered to tubes without an anticoagulant.
14. First, he or she must be completely familiar with all of the equipment and well-versed in all blood collecting procedures. Second, the phlebotomist must be able to follow directions quickly and correctly.

# CHAPTER 6
1. d
2. b, c, d
3. b, c
4. a, b, c, d, e
5. b
6. b, c, d
7. a, b, c

# CHAPTER 7
1. Manuals, procedures (technical, administrative, safety, quality control), continuing education, staff meetings, performance evaluations, memoranda, and bulletin boards.
2. Be consistent in format and headings; allow enough space for patient descriptions, print-outs, imprints, or handwriting; have adequate number of copies; make it clear and concise; be convenient to handle, store, sort, and attach to a patient's chart.
3. Hand delivered, hospital transportation department, pneumatic tube system.
4. Medical records, staff on inpatient floors, laboratory, hospital business office.
5. Test requisitioning.
6. On-line computer input of test request information by the requesting authority is the most error-free method because computer systems have the capability of performing automatic checks on the input.
7. Correct and proper identification of the patient should be made prior to obtaining the specimen.

# CHAPTER 8

1. A. Greet the patient
   b. Identify yourself
   c. Ask the patient's name
   d. Ask the patient's address. Required by some hospitals
   e. Check the laboratory request slip with the patient's I.D. number on his/her wristband.
   f. Label the tube of blood before leaving the patient's bedside.
2. a. Have the patient apply pressure to the venipuncture site.
   b. After the labeling the tube(s) check the condition of the site and general condition of the patient.
   c. Observe the patient after he/she stands up to make sure there are no adverse signs (fainting, bleeding).
3. a. Malaria
   b. Hepatitis
   c. Herpes
   d. Tuberculosis
   e. Syphilis
   f. AIDS
4. The patient has the right to:
   a. Considerate and respectful care.
   b. Know who is performing a procedure and what the procedure is.
   c. Refuse treatment.
   d. Privacy of person, treatment.
   e. Privacy of method and condition of payment.
   f. Reasonable service.
   g. Continuity of care.
   h. Know what rules are important to his/her care (instructions for preparation of patient for laboratory testing normally given by phlebotomist).
   i. An environment free of conflict.
5. a. Sigmund Freud
   b. Abraham Maslow
   c. Douglas McGregor
   d. Frederick Herzberg
6. Maslow's hierarchy of needs is: physiologic, safety, love, esteem, and self actualization.
7. Theory X is based on the statement that people prefer to be directed, have an inherent dislike of work. Also they must be coerced, controlled, and threatened to get them to work.
8. Theory Y is based on the premise that mankind wants to work, will seek responsibility, and will exercise self-direction.
9. In *civil law*, one person sues another person (this can be a company, hospital, etc.). In *criminal law* the government (city, state, or federal) brings suit against a person for breaking a statute or law.

10. The expected performance of health-care personnel are generally expressed in standards of behavior or performance.

## CHAPTER 9
1. a, b
2. b, c, d
3. b, c, d
4. c, d
5. a, b, d

## CHAPTER 10
1. a. source and number of patients
   b. age and/or sex of patients
   c. socioeconomic or ethnic background of patients
   d. proportion of ambulatory patients to bed patients
   e. the location of the phlebotomy unit
   f. availability of a computer
2. a. draw or collect specimens as required by physicians
   b. provide a liaison service between the physicians and the laboratory
   c. deliver specimens to appropriate section and communicate results promptly
   d. under direction of physician or nurse to aid in delivery of patient care as required
3. a. volume of specimens
   b. permanent assignment or daily flexible assignments
   c. number of times that collections will be made
   d. other duties in addition to specimen collection
   e. the special nature of the patient population
4. a, c
5. a. understanding
   b. respect for others
   c. knowledge of situation
   d. adaptability
   e. enthusiasm
   f. objectivity
   g. communication skills
   h. confidence in oneself and one's subordinates
   i. proper use of authority
   j. providing recognition .
6. a. number of critical care areas
   b. time of delivery of food service
   c. time of first surgery scheduled
   d. emergency or trauma center patients

7. a. volume of specimens and other work anticipated
   b. human hours required and level of skills needed
   c. materials and outside services
   d. equipment
   e. revenue and rate setting
8. 5.34 FTE
   $3800 \times 12 = 45,600$
   $5000 \times \ \ 6 = 30,000$
   $\ \ 100 \times 10 = \ \ 1,000$
   $\ \ \ \ 50 \times \ \ 6 = \ \ \ \ 300$

   76,900 CAP units (min) $\div$ 60 = 1281.6 hours
   There are paid workhours over an 8-hour shift in a 30-day month of
   240 paid hours. 1281.6 $\div$ 240 = 5.43 FTE
9. See Table 10.2
   The labor would be double $-$ \$1.08
   The collecting tube would be .05
   No tourniquet, no needle but a lancet at about same cost
   Therefore total cost would be \$1.43.
10. a. to evaluate progress of unit
    b. to evaluate personnel performance
    c. to identify adjustments that need to be made
    d. to fulfill responsibility for equipment and supplies
11. c
12. c
13. b
14. d
15. b
16. a
17. d
18. b
19. d
20. a

# Index